Contemporary Diagnosis and Management of

Parkinson's Disease®

Kathleen M. Shannon, MD
Associate Professor
Department of Neurological Sciences
Section of Movement Disorders
Rush University Medical Center
Chicago, Illinois

Foreword by
Ray L. Watts, MD
Chairman, Department of Neurology
University of Alabama-Birmingham
Birmingham, Alabama

First Edition

Published by Handbooks in Health Care Co.,
Newtown, Pennsylvania, USA

This book has been prepared and is presented as a service to the medical community. The information provided reflects the knowledge, experience, and personal opinions of the author, Kathleen M. Shannon, MD, Associate Professor, Department of Neurological Sciences, Section of Movement Disorders, Rush University Medical Center, Chicago, Illinois.

This book is not intended to replace or to be used as a substitute for the complete prescribing information prepared by each manufacturer for each drug. Because of possible variations in drug indications, in dosage information, in newly described toxicities, in drug/drug interactions, and in other items of importance, reference to such complete prescribing information is definitely recommended before any of the drugs discussed are used or prescribed.

International Standard Book Number: 978-1-884065-72-9

Library of Congress Catalog Card Number: 2007933639

First Edition

Table of Contents

Foreword

In recent years, our understanding and knowledge regarding Parkinson's disease (PD) has greatly advanced. It is now recognized as a multifaceted disease, with nonmotor features causing as much or even greater disability than the classic motor features. While slowness of movement, muscle rigidity and stiffness, postural and gait abnormalities, and tremor are significant causes of everyday disability, the neuropsychiatric features of PD, ie, depression, anxiety, hallucinations, psychosis, and dementia, are of even greater concern to many patients and their families.

Autonomic dysfunction is wide ranging, and may be exacerbated by the medications used to treat the primary and/or secondary symptoms of PD, eg, orthostatic hypotension, constipation, urinary urgency and frequency, and erectile dysfunction (ED) in males. Sleep abnormalities are myriad in PD, especially in the advanced stages of the disease, and they have been under-recognized and underappreciated until recently.

Knowledge related to the underlying biochemical pathophysiology of PD continues to advance, and we now have a broad range of antiparkinsonian medications that allow the effective control for many years of motor symptoms (and some nonmotor symptoms) in most patients. For patients with motor complications, such as dyskinesias and wearing-off fluctuations, that result from long-term treatment with levodopa and other dopaminergic therapies, deep-brain stimulation surgery can be life changing in appropriate settings.

Dr. Kathleen Shannon has done an excellent job of covering the wide spectrum of topics now relevant to a modern understanding of PD, and the breadth and depth of her knowledge is evident in the logically organized range of chapters featured in this handbook. Moreover, her approach is straightforward, and the knowledge presented about PD is practical. This handbook should be very helpful for health-care professionals, and even the well-informed public of this era will find it to be written in a clear and understandable manner. I recommend it enthusiastically and congratulate Dr. Shannon for sharing her knowledge in such a user-friendly and informative format.

Ray L. Watts, MD
John N. Whitaker Professor and
Chairman, Department of Neurology
University of Alabama at Birmingham
Birmingham, Alabama

Chapter 1

Introduction, Epidemiology, and Scope of the Problem

P arkinsonism was first described by James Parkinson in 1817. His astute presentation of case histories defined a syndrome characterized by tremor, bradykinesia, and postural reflex impairment.[1] Charcot described the characteristic rigidity and named the disorder Parkinson's disease (PD) about 60 years after Parkinson's monograph was published. Although the specific pathologic basis of the disease was elucidated in 1919,[2] clinicians only began to understand the biochemical basis of PD around 1960.[3] The discovery of decreased dopamine in the brains of patients with PD led to the successful use of high doses of levodopa in the mid-1960s.[4]

Definition

Parkinsonism is a symptom complex that includes tremor, bradykinesia, rigidity, and postural reflex impairment (Table 1-1). Several tremor types are seen in parkinsonism. The classic rest tremor of parkinsonism affects the jaw, facial muscles or tongue, or the limbs. The tremor frequency ranges from 4 to 6 cycles/sec. In the limbs, pronation/supination movements of the wrist and flexion/extension movements of the fingers are common. The combination of these movements led clinicians to describe the tremor as 'pill rolling.' The tremor improves or disappears with movement, but may recur when the patient assumes a new posture. The presence of this type of rest tremor is highly suggestive of parkinsonism, specifically PD. Other

Table 1-1: Cardinal Signs of Parkinsonism

- Tremor
- Rigidity
- Bradykinesia
- Postural reflex impairment

tremors are also commonly seen in parkinsonism. Posture-holding tremor and tremor that is most prominent at the end of movement trajectory occur with greater frequency than rest tremor in parkinsonism. Unfortunately, postural and action tremor are not specific signs of parkinsonism and are more often seen in patients with essential tremor or physiologic tremor enhanced by drugs or metabolic states. Bradykinesia describes several abnormalities of motor function, including difficulty initiating movement, slowness, reduced range, and difficulty with repetitive movements. It can reduce the range of facial expression and lead to soft or hypophonic speech, drooling, loss of spontaneous movements (ie, shifting in a chair, crossing and uncrossing the legs), lack of associated movements (ie, arm swing), and slowing of gait with shortening of the stride. When assessing bradykinesia, the clinician should observe spontaneous patient movements and ask the patient to perform several repetitive tasks, such as tapping the thumb with the index finger, clenching and releasing the fists, making pronation/supination wrist movements, and tapping the toes or stamping the heels. The clinician should assess the speed and amplitude of the movements. To assess rigidity, passively move the neck, arms, and legs to assess the degree of resistance. The rigidity of parkinsonism is generally present throughout the range of motion and in both flexors and extensors. Unlike gegenhalten or paratonic rigidity, it does not increase as the speed of movement in-

Table 1-2: Other Signs of Parkinsonism

- Decreased smiling and blinking
- Drooling
- Soft voice
- Slow thinking
- Micrographia
- Difficulty buttoning buttons
- Difficulty with repetitive activities (tooth brushing)
- Feeling of weakness
- Dragging the leg
- Tightness, stiffness, achiness
- Stooped posture
- Generalized slowing of activity
- Deterioration in golf or tennis game
- Sleep disorder
- Difficulty initiating walking
- Freezing

creases. The rigidity of parkinsonism may be felt constantly during the movement ('lead pipe' rigidity) or may increase and decrease with a ratcheting quality ('cogwheel' rigidity). To assess postural reflex impairment in parkinsonism, ask the patient to stand with his or her feet about a shoulder width apart. Warn the patient that he or she will be pulled off balance, and ask that he or she try to maintain balance. Then, pull back on the patient's shoulders with enough force to pull him or her off balance. Record the response. A normal person will take a step back to recover balance.

A parkinsonian patient with mild postural reflex impairment may take several steps to recover. The examiner may have to catch the patient with moderate impairment so he or she will not fall. Severely affected patients will fall spontaneously. Postural reflex impairment is not specific for the diagnosis of parkinsonism because it occurs with several types of motor and sensory dysfunction. The presence of two of the four cardinal signs is sufficient to make the diagnosis of parkinsonism. Patients with parkinsonism complain of many other symptoms, which are listed in Table 1-2.

Many symptoms and signs of parkinsonism are normally associated with aging. We expect our elders to be shakier, slower, and less spontaneous with their movements, to walk with a short stride and shuffling footsteps, and to be unsteady. Indeed, formal studies confirm that the symptoms and signs of parkinsonism increase with age. In a community-based study of East Boston residents, the prevalence of parkinsonism was 30% for people between ages 75 and 84, and 52% for persons older than age 85. Whether these features represent normal aging of the central nervous system (CNS) or reflect one or more underrecognized acquired structural pathologies or degenerative processes remains undetermined. However, the importance of parkinsonian signs in the elderly is underscored by the author's finding that the presence of parkinsonism is associated with an overall risk of death twice that of unaffected persons.[5]

The motor features of parkinsonism result from a decrease in dopamine neurotransmission in the nigrostriatal pathway. The cell bodies of the nigrostriatal dopamine system are in the substantia nigra of the midbrain. Their axons project to the caudate nucleus and putamen, which together form the striatum (Figure 1-1). Decreased dopamine neurotransmission may be caused by disease or dysfunction of the presynaptic neuron in the midbrain substantia nigra, reducing the amount of dopamine available to striatal dopamine receptors. Some examples of presynaptic parkinsonism are PD, structural disease in

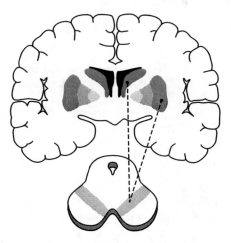

Postsynaptic Parkinsonism
- Atypical parkinsonism
- Structural lesion of striatum
- Dopamine receptor blockade

Presynaptic Parkinsonism
- Parkinson's disease (PD)
- Structural lesion
  of substantia nigra
- Impaired synthesis/release
  of dopamine

Figure 1-1: Etiologies of parkinsonism. The nigrostriatal dopaminergic pathway. Dopaminergic cells have their bodies in the substantia nigra (pars compacta) and their axons synapse on cells in the caudate nucleus and putamen (striatum). Parkinsonism may result from disease or dysfunction of cells in the substantia nigra (presynaptic parkinsonism) or of cells in the striatum (postsynaptic parkinsonism).

the midbrain, or disorders of the metabolic pathway for dopamine. Parkinsonism may also result from disorders at the postsynaptic level in the striatum. Some examples of postsynaptic parkinsonism are degenerative conditions affecting striatal neurons, such as the atypical parkinsonisms; acquired focal striatal lesions, such as infarction and neurotoxic damage; and pharmacologic blockade of the postsynaptic dopamine receptor (Figure 1-1).

Epidemiology

About 80% of parkinsonism cases seen in a neurologic practice relate to PD, which is second to Alzheimer's disease (AD) among degenerative CNS disorders of aging. PD is rare before age 50 and increases dramatically with age thereafter. The prevalence of PD has been variably estimated as 20 to 180/100,000 persons.[6] A summary of data from population-based studies in seven European countries suggested the overall prevalence of PD in persons older than age 65 was 1.8%, ranging from 0.6% for persons aged 65 to 69 years to 2.6% of persons aged 85 to 89 years.[7] Postmortem studies suggest as many as 10% of 70-year-olds have pathologic changes of early PD at death.[8] This is clearly not enough to account for the overwhelming appearance of parkinsonian signs in the aging population, but does suggest that a significant number of patients may escape disease detection or may be in the presymptomatic phase of the illness at death. An increase in disease prevalence over the past several decades relates to an aging population and to postponing death in affected persons by highly effective symptomatic treatment. With demographic changes that call for an increase in the number of the elderly in the population worldwide, the prevalence of PD can be expected to increase.[9]

The influences of gender and race on disease incidence remain unclear. In subspecialty clinic-based series, men make up 60% of patients and the overwhelming majority of patients are white. The incidence of PD is greater in men than in women. In Olmsted County, Minnesota, the estimated mean annual incidence was 12.4 cases/100,000 women and 16.2 cases/100,000 men.[10] However, in some population-based cohorts, prevalence does not differ significantly between women and men.[7] Cultural factors may contribute to the perceived gender inequity in PD. In a study of referral patterns from primary care providers to neurologists or PD subspecialty clinics, women were less likely to receive subspecialty care than men.[11]

Two studies reporting race-specific PD incidence found rates similar among African-American men, Asian-American men, and American men of European origin.[12,13] However, studies have found a reduced prevalence of PD among African-American and Asian-American men, suggesting reduced ascertainment or poorer survival in these populations.[12,13]

Epidemiologic studies have failed to identify a prominent genetic or environmental etiology for typical PD. It is likely that, in most cases, the etiology of PD reflects an interaction between genetic and environmental influences. Although about 30% of patients with clinically typical PD have a positive family history,[14] <5% have a pedigree suggesting dominant inheritance of the condition. A number of genetic factors have recently been identified in familial PD. In a small number of people with dominantly inherited parkinsonism, mutations in the α-synuclein gene have been reported (PARK1; chromosome 4q21-4q23). The resulting parkinsonism resembles sporadic PD, although earlier onset and more prominent autonomic, affective, and behavior changes have been reported. In other families, duplication or triplication of the α-synuclein gene has been associated with parkinsonism and dementia, respectively (PARK4; chromosome 4p15). A German family with autosomal-dominant PD has been found to have a mutation in the ubiquitin carboxy-terminal hydrolase L1 gene (PARK5; chromosome 4p14). There is increasing interest in another locus in dominantly inherited PD. This locus maps to the

12th chromosome and is related to dominantly inherited PD with incomplete penetrance. Mutations in this gene, leucine-rich repeat kinase 2 (LRRK2), appear common in patients of North African and Ashkenazi origin (PARK8; chromosome 12p11.2-q13.1). Some patients with recessively inherited early-onset levodopa-responsive parkinsonism have been found to have mutations in the parkin gene (PARK2; chromosome 6q25.2-27). These mutations may be detected in as many as half of all PD cases with onset before age 40 and an autosomal-recessive inheritance pattern. Mutations in the phosphatase and tensin homolog (PTEN)-induced kinase 1 (PINK1) gene have also been identified in some families with recessively inherited PD (PARK6; chromosome 1p36). Another recessively inherited parkinsonism has been related to mutations in the DJ1 gene (PARK7; chromosome 1p36). While these genetic discoveries have done much to advance our knowledge of the etiology and pathogenesis of PD, there is as yet no role for routine genetic testing in PD.[15]

The risk of developing PD when a parent is affected is three to four times higher than the risk in the population at large. In a large study of PD in male twins, concordance rates were similar in monozygotic and dizygotic twin pairs with onset of parkinsonism after age 50. In cases where the disease began before age 50, concordance in monozygotic twins was much higher than in dizygotic twins, suggesting a prominent genetic component.[16] In addition, using positron emission tomography (PET) measures of presynaptic dopamine function, a progressive decline can be demonstrated in monozygotic co-twins of PD patients, suggesting concordance although the co-twin may not have reached the threshold of symptomatic PD.[17] Thus, clinicians believe there may be strong genetic factors influencing the development of parkinsonism or PD in a small number of families who inherit the disease in an autosomal-dominant or autosomal-recessive pattern especially with early-onset PD. A modest genetic contribution may exist in patients with the typical sporadically appearing form of the illness.

The argument for an environmental etiology of PD rests on several lines of evidence, including its relative rarity before industrialization, the late onset of the disease, and certain epidemiologic associations. Pure environmental etiologies for parkinsonism have been identified. The most compelling is the acute, severe parkinsonism that followed systemic exposure to 1-methyl-4-phenyl-1,2,3,6-tetrahydropyridine (MPTP) in a small number of patients who abused a designer narcotic in California.[18] Similarities between MPTP and other putative endogenous and environmental neurotoxins, such as tetrahydroisoquinoline and β-carboline derivatives, raise intriguing possibilities about the disease etiology, but there remains no proof of a link between the disease and a specific neurotoxin.[19] Other environmental etiologies for parkinsonism include manganese, Guamanian cycad fruit, and viral infections.[20]

A number of epidemiologic studies show a link between PD and environmental insults, including head trauma, rural living, well-water drinking, and exposure to pesticides.[21] No single environmental culprit has been identified by these studies. Cigarette smoking has been shown to be negatively associated with the likelihood of developing PD,[21] but this may partially reflect premorbid personality traits that lead future disease sufferers to eschew such habits[22] or the effects of competitive mortality.[23]

PD is considered a disorder with both genetic and environmental influences. It is best thought of as a clinical spectrum with purely genetic forms on one end and purely environmental forms on the other.

Scope of the Problem

In the era before symptomatic treatment with levodopa, severe disability or death occurred in 28% of PD patients by 5 years of disease, 61% of patients by 10 years, and 83% of patients by 15 years of disease.[24] The introduction of levodopa was associated with a 50% reduction in PD mortality and dramatically reduced disability. Fifteen years after the introduction of levodopa, only 9% of PD patients were severely disabled or dead by 5 years, 21% by 10 years, and 38% by 15 years.[25] However, the mortality of PD remains elevated. In a recent Danish study that included 345 subjects, standard mortality was 1.7 for men and 2.5 for women. The usual causes of death in PD are respiratory tract infection or failure, cardiac failure, and carcinoma.[26] In the United States, PD now accounts for the loss of 36,000 years of life and 447,000 disability-adjusted life years annually. PD patients use 162,000 hospital days annually.[27] Patients with PD, particularly women, are at increased risk of hip fracture, and have a greater residual morbidity after fracture when compared with elderly control patients.[28] In a prospective study in Olmsted County, Minnesota, 27% of PD patients sustained new hip fractures within 10 years of diagnosis of PD.[29] PD patients make up nearly 7% of all nursing home residents.[30] Nursing home placement is generally permanent and associated with a high mortality rate.[31,32]

Virtually every measure of quality of life and economic burden is influenced by PD. Consistent associations exist between increasing severity of illness and declines in functional status, well being, and overall health-related quality of life. By the time PD is moderate in severity, 78% of patients are unable to perform one or more daily activities, and 50% are retired or unemployed because of the disease.[33]

References

1. Parkinson J: *An Essay on the Shaking Palsy*. London, Whittingham and Rowland, 1817.

2. Tretiakoff C: *Contribution a l'Etude de l'Anatomie du Locus Niger.* These de Paris, Paris, 1919.

3. Barbeau A: Biochemistry of Parkinson's disease. International Congress Series 348, 1961:152-153.

4. Hornykiewicz O: Dopamine (3-hydroxytyramine) and brain function. *Pharmacol Rev* 1966;18:925-964.

5.   Bennett DA, Beckett LA, Murray AM, et al: Prevalence of parkinsonian signs and associated mortality in a community population of older people (see comments). *N Engl J Med* 1996;334:71-76.

6.   Schoenberg BS: Descriptive epidemiology of Parkinson's disease: disease distribution and hypothesis formulation. *Adv Neurol* 1987;45:277-283.

7.   de Rijk M, Launer LJ, Berger K, et al: Prevalence of Parkinson's disease in Europe: A collaborative study of population-based cohorts. Neurologic Diseases in the Elderly Research Group. *Neurology* 2000;54:S21-S23.

8.   Fearnley JM, Lees AJ: Ageing and Parkinson's disease: substantia nigra regional selectivity. *Brain* 1991;114:2283-2301.

9.   Dorsey ER, Constantinescu R, Thompson JP, et al: Projected number of people with Parkinson disease in the most populous nations, 2005 through 2030. *Neurology* 2007;68:384-386.

10.   Tanner CM, Thelen JA, Offord KP, et al: Parkinson's disease incidence in Olmsted County, MN: 1935-1988. *Neurology* 1992;42(suppl 3):194.

11.   Rybicki BA, Johnson CC, Gorell JM: Demographic differences in referral rates to neurologists of patients with suspected Parkinson's disease: implications for case-control study design. *Neuroepidemiology* 1995;14:72-81.

12.   Morens DM, Davis JW, Grandinetti A, et al: Epidemiologic observations on Parkinson's disease: incidence and mortality in a prospective study of middle-aged men. *Neurology* 1996;46:1044-1050.

13.   Mayeux R, Marder K, Cote LJ, et al: The frequency of idiopathic Parkinson's disease by age, ethnic group, and sex in northern Manhattan, 1988-1993 (see comments). *Am J Epidemiol* 1995;142:820-827.

14.   Marder K, Tang MX, Mejia H, et al: Risk of Parkinson's disease among first-degree relatives: A community-based study. *Neurology* 1996;47:155-160.

15.   Tan EK, Jankovic J: Genetic testing in Parkinson disease: promises and pitfalls. *Arch Neurol* 2006;63:1232-1237.

16.   Tanner CM, Ottman R, Goldman SM, et al: Parkinson disease in twins: an etiologic study. *JAMA* 1999;281:341-346.

17.   Piccini P, Brooks DJ: Etiology of Parkinson's disease: contributions from 18F-DOPA positron emission tomography. *Adv Neurol* 1999;80:227-231.

18. Langston JW, Ballard P: Parkinsonism induced by 1-methyl-4-phenyl-1,2,3,6-tetrahydropyridine (MPTP): implications for treatment and the pathogenesis of Parkinson's disease. *Can J Neurol Sci* 1984;11:160-165.

19. Mizuno Y, Shimoda-Matsubayashi S, Matsumine H, et al: Genetic and environmental factors in the pathogenesis of Parkinson's disease. *Adv Neurol* 1999;80:171-179.

20. Williams AC, Smith ML, Waring RH, et al: Idiopathic Parkinson's disease: A genetic and environmental model. *Adv Neurol* 1999;80:215-218.

21. Chade AR, Kasten M, Tanner CM: Nongenetic causes of Parkinson's disease. *J Neural Transm Suppl* 2006;(70):147-151.

22. Todes CJ, Lees AJ: The pre-morbid personality of patients with Parkinson's disease. *J Neurol Neurosurg Psychiatry* 1985;48:97-100.

23. Morens DM, Grandinetti A, Reed D, et al: Cigarette smoking and protection from Parkinson's disease: false association or etiologic clue? *Neurology* 1995;45:1041-1051.

24. Hoehn MM, Yahr MD: Parkinsonism: onset, progression and mortality. *Neurology* 1967;17:427-442.

25. Hoehn MM: Parkinsonism treated with levodopa: progression and mortality. In: Birkmayer W, Duvoisin RC, eds: *Extrapyramidal Disorders*. New York, NY, Springer-Verlag, 1983, pp 253-264.

26. Roos RA, Jongen JC, van der Velde EA: Clinical course of patients with idiopathic Parkinson's disease. *Mov Disord* 1996;11:236-242.

27. Gross CP, Anderson GF, Powe NR: The relation between funding by the National Institutes of Health and the burden of disease. *N Engl J Med* 1999;340:1881-1887.

28. Hammer AJ: Intertrochanteric and femoral neck fractures in patients with parkinsonism. *S Afr Med J* 1991;79:200-202.

29. Johnell O, Melton LJ, Atkinson EJ, et al: Fracture risk in patients with parkinsonism: a population-based study in Olmsted County, Minnesota. *Age Ageing* 1992;21:32-38.

30. Mitchell SL, Kiely DK, Kiel DP, et al: The epidemiology, clinical characteristics, and natural history of older nursing home residents with a diagnosis of Parkinson's disease. *J Am Geriatr Soc* 1996;44:394-399.

31. Goetz CG, Stebbins GT: Mortality and hallucinations in nursing home patients with advanced Parkinson's disease. *Neurology* 1995; 45:669-671.

32. Goetz CG, Stebbins GT: Risk factors for nursing home placement in advanced Parkinson's disease. *Neurology* 1993;43: 2227-2229.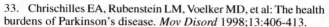

33. Chrischilles EA, Rubenstein LM, Voelker MD, et al: The health burdens of Parkinson's disease. *Mov Disord* 1998;13:406-413.

Diagnosis and Differential Diagnosis

C linicians make the diagnosis of parkinsonism when they find two of the four cardinal signs as discussed in Chapter 2. Unfortunately, there is no objective way to diagnose parkinsonism, and the misdiagnosis and underdiagnosis rates can be substantial. For example, in a study where 402 persons taking antiparkinsonian drugs were identified through pharmacy records, only 74% were found to have parkinsonism.[1] Once the diagnosis of parkinsonism is established, the next step is to differentiate between Parkinson's disease (PD) and the other forms of parkinsonism. Clinicians must make this distinction because PD has well understood pathophysiology and pharmacology, as well as a predictable response to medications and prognosis. Other forms of parkinsonism respond poorly to antiparkinsonian medications, and have more rapidly progressive disability and higher mortality. In the aforementioned study, only 54% of patients taking antiparkinsonian drugs were found to meet the clinical criteria for probable PD.[1] The differential diagnosis of parkinsonism is listed in Table 2-1.

Parkinson's Disease

PD is a presynaptic disease defined by its pathologic appearance. It is characterized by degeneration of pigmented dopaminergic neurons in the substantia nigra pars compacta (SNpc). Cut sections of the midbrain in patients with PD show pallor of the substantia nigra, which is apparent to the naked eye. Lewy bodies are acidophilic inclusions, which are spherical and have a dense core and peripheral halo, are seen in the neuronal cytoplasm of the substantia nigra and other pigmented brainstem nuclei.[2]

Positron emission tomography (PET) scanning using fluorodopa accurately identifies patients with the presynaptic dopamine deficit associated with PD, but is not clinically available. Several single-photon emission computerized tomography ligands that label components of the presynaptic dopamine terminal appear to accurately identify the presynaptic dopamine deficiency associated with PD.[3] However, these will not be clinically available soon.

For now, the diagnosis of PD rests on clinical criteria. Unfortunately, clinicopathologic studies suggest that the clinician's impression of PD is often wrong. In a large clinicopathologic study, the clinician's impression of PD was confirmed pathologically only 76% of the time.[4] Diagnoses in the other patients included progressive supranuclear palsy (PSP), Alzheimer's disease (AD), multiple system atrophy, vascular disease, isolated substantia nigra atrophy, postencephalitic parkinsonism, and normal findings. Diagnostic criteria for PD have been proposed. While these criteria increase the specificity of clinical diagnosis, they decrease its sensitivity.[4] The most commonly used research clinical diagnostic criteria for PD are: asymmetry of signs at onset, the presence of two or more cardinal signs including rest tremor, and a substantial improvement on levodopa treatment sustained for 1 year. Using these criteria, the specificity of diagnosis is about 90%, but about 30% of PD cases are falsely excluded.[5] Tables 2-2 and 2-3 list clinical criteria that increase and decrease, respectively, the likelihood that a patient will have pathologic changes of PD at autopsy. Although some of these signs may be obvious early in the disease course, some patients will evolve more atypical features, making periodic reassessment of the diagnosis prudent.

Table 2-1: Differential Diagnosis of Parkinsonism

Neurodegenerative Disease

- Parkinson's disease (PD)
- Atypical parkinsonism
  - Progressive supranuclear palsy (PSP)
  - Multiple system atrophy (MSA)
    - Striatonigral degeneration type (MSA-parkinsonism)
    - Autonomic type (Shy-Drager syndrome) (MSA-autonomic)
    - Olivopontocerebellar atrophy type (MSA-cerebellar)
  - Corticobasal degeneration (CBD)
- Alzheimer's disease (AD) with extrapyramidal signs
- Diffuse Lewy body disease (DLBD)
- Huntington's disease (HD) (Westphal variant)
- Wilson's disease (WD)
- Pantothenate-kinase-associated neurodegeneration (PKAN)
- Calcification of the basal ganglia
- Creutzfeldt-Jakob disease (CJD)

Clinical diagnostic criteria are important for defining homogeneous patient groups for clinical trials and other research studies and may help physicians focus on the salient features of the illness. However, optimal treatment of this population is probably favored by a more relaxed approach to diagnosis.

Acquired Structural Disease
- Subcortical vascular disease
- Calcification of the basal ganglia
- Hydrocephalus
- Brain tumor
- Subdural hematoma
- Anoxic brain injury
- Traumatic brain injury
- Toxic brain injury
  - Carbon monoxide poisoning
  - Manganese intoxication
  - MPTP-induced parkinsonism
  - Cyanide poisoning
  - Carbon disulfide poisoning
  - Methanol intoxication

Metabolic Causes
- Drug-induced parkinsonism (DIP)
  - Dopamine receptor blockers
  - Other drugs

MPTP=1-methyl-4-phenyl-1,2,3,6-tetrahydropyridine

Temporal evolution of PD and its treatment

The symptoms and signs of PD usually begin unilaterally. Tremor at rest or decreased fine motor dexterity are the usual presenting complaints. Handwriting becomes small and cramped (micrographia), buttoning buttons may be slower, and repetitive movements associated

23

Table 2-2: Signs That Increase the Likelihood of PD

- Unilateral onset
- Rest tremor
- Levodopa responsiveness
- Asymmetric progression
- Clinical course lasting ≥10 years
- Motor response fluctuations
- Levodopa-induced dyskinesia

with brushing teeth or washing the body may be slow and laborious. Poorly localized pain in the shoulder or arm leads to the diagnosis of bursitis or arthritis in some patients. Some patients present with decreased arm swing when walking, or limp or drag their legs. Speech disorder, postural flexion, or impaired postural reflexes when falling are less common presentations and may reflect more widespread degenerative changes associated with other neurodegenerative disorders (see below). Some patients first notice symptoms following a minor trauma, surgical procedure, or stress. In others, the onset of symptoms is hard to pinpoint, and some patients are described by their spouses as 'always slower than others.' In a well-documented case of PD occurring in a famous soccer player, subtle physical signs existed at least 14 years before diagnosis and physical abnormalities were discernible on game videotapes as long as 8 years before he sought medical attention.[6] The asymmetry of signs and symptoms frequently leads the clinician to consider stroke or brain tumor, radiculopathy, or peripheral neuropathy. Before a diagnosis of PD, many patients have symptoms of depression, excessive daytime sleepiness, or constipation.[7,8] Neuroimaging studies and electromyography (EMG) are frequently performed at this stage and found to be normal.

As the disease progresses, it may create some midline symptoms including reduced facial expression and mild rounding of the shoulders. Speech can become softer and more slurred. Symptoms become apparent on the contralateral side, although the side initially involved remains more prominently affected throughout the disease. Most patients have been diagnosed by this time and are on therapy. In the 5 years after antiparkinsonian therapy begins, patients usually do well. Most continue working, driving, and maintaining their usual activities, including sports. The next 5 years are often characterized by nuisance symptoms and side effects. Medication response may become less predictable, and complications of antiparkinsonian therapy, such as drug-induced involuntary movements, can become apparent. Many patients have disordered sleep or altered dream phenomena. Some patients may hallucinate. Most patients have one or more motor complications between 10 and 15 years of therapy. Most take at least two antiparkinsonian medications, and many stop working or give up driving. Most complain about cognition or memory lapses. Sleep and dreams become more abnormal. Hallucinations are more frequent. Gait tends to deteriorate. Gait initiation may be slow, a phenomenon known as start hesitation. Gait may also slow or suddenly freeze in visually crowded environments, or when the patient experiences many confusing sensory stimuli. Falling is more common. Most patients give up driving and physical recreational activities and often rely on others for some activities of daily living. Swallowing and speech become more troublesome. Some patients complain about disordered sweating and orthostatic dizziness, and most have urinary problems and constipation. After 15 to 20 years of therapy, as many as two thirds of PD patients have died or are severely disabled.[9] Nearly all surviving

Table 2-3: Signs That Decrease the Likelihood of PD

Atypical Onset or Course

- Symmetric onset
- Early gait disability or falling
- Severe disability within 5 years
- Stepwise progression
- Sustained remission

Atypical Clinical Features

- Supranuclear gaze palsy
- Cerebellar signs
- Babinski's sign
- Lower motor neuron signs
- Oculogyric crises
- Early dementia
- Early autonomic impairment
- Involuntary gasping respirations
- Stridor
- Sleep apnea

patients say their medication is unpredictable, and most show some evidence of medication-related complications. The medication schedule itself may be complicated with short interdose intervals (1 to 3 hours) and multiple medications. Most patients complain about gait, including start hesitation, poor turning, freezing, or falling. Dysphagia and weight loss are common. Assistance with the activities of daily living is usually required, and many patients depend on walkers or wheelchairs. Many show signs of dementia.

Another Etiology Likely
(Symptomatic Parkinsonism)

- Strokes
- Repeated head injury
- More than one affected relative
- Neuroleptic exposure
- Toxic exposure (eg, manganese, MPTP, carbon monoxide)
- Tumor
- Hydrocephalus

MPTP=1-methyl-4-phenyl-1,2,3,6-tetrahydropyridine

Among patients with early-onset PD, many retain some independence, but few work, drive, or engage in physical recreation activities. Medication schedules are complex and include many drugs for parkinsonism and treatment-related complications. Sleep disruption is common, and many patients have altered dream phenomena (ie, drug-induced hallucinations or psychosis). Depression is a common complication of PD at all stages of the illness, affecting about 40% of patients.

Table 2-4: The Hoehn and Yahr Staging System for PD[12]

Stage 1	Unilateral signs and symptoms
Stage 2	Bilateral signs and symptoms, postural reflexes preserved
Stage 3	Bilateral signs and symptoms, impaired postural reflexes, moderate disability
Stage 4	Severe gait disability, able to stand and walk unassisted
Stage 5	Unable to stand or walk unassisted, bed- or wheelchair-bound state

Several studies of the natural history of PD show that its natural progression rate varies greatly between patients, but is fairly consistent within patients. However, the progression rate appears to slow after 9 or 10 years, and the clinician can have a fairly good idea how disability will progress by assessing disease severity and response to medication at the 5-year point. Identified risk factors for faster disease progression include older age at onset, predominance of akinesia and rigidity over tremor, and cognitive decline.[10,11]

For the purposes of clinical research, PD was divided into five stages.[12] Stage 1 is characterized by unilateral signs and symptoms, Stage 2 by bilateral signs and symptoms without postural reflex impairment, Stage 3 by bilateral symptoms with postural reflex impairment and moderate disability, Stage 4 by severe gait disability with retained independence for standing and walking, and Stage 5 by the bed- or wheelchair-bound state (Table 2-4).

An awareness of the evolution of the disease helps the clinician both recognize the disease in its later stages and differentiate between disease-related symptoms and those related to pharmacotherapy.

Other Important Degenerative Causes of Parkinsonism

Progressive supranuclear palsy

Progressive supranuclear palsy (PSP) is a rare disorder of midlife characterized by parkinsonism with prominent gait disorder, supranuclear gaze palsy, pseudobulbar dysfunction, and behavior changes. The age-adjusted prevalence is 6.4/100,000 people.[13] Although some familial cases have been reported, genetic factors do not seem important in most cases.[14] The condition most often begins with gait instability and falling. Judgment is impaired, and patients engage in risky or unsafe activities, such as climbing ladders or trees, even when cautioned not to do so. Parkinsonian signs are usually symmetric, and rest tremor is rare. Volitional extraocular movements are impaired, primarily for downgaze. While the patient with PSP has difficulty initiating eye movements, a full range of extraocular movements can be elicited by having the patient focus on a fixed object and moving the head up and down and from side to side. Abnormal eyelid movements, including involuntary eye closure and impaired volitional eye opening, are present. The patient's facial expression appears worried or startled rather than flat and expressionless as is seen in PD. Speech is dysarthric and has a strained quality. Dysphagia and aspiration are prominent. Frontal-lobe-type personality is common.[15] Some patients with PSP have pure akinesia or a parkinsonian syndrome without extraocular muscle impairment. PSP can also present as an isolated dementia. Neuroimaging studies show enlargement of the third ventricle with atrophy of the lower midbrain and thinning of the quadrigeminal plate.[16] PSP patients respond only modestly to antiparkinsonian drugs, and toxicity is common.[17] The condition progresses rapidly with a median duration of 3.1 years at the time assisted ambulation is necessary, and 8.2 years when a wheelchair is required. The median disease duration at death is 9.7 years.[18]

Multiple system atrophy

Multiple system atrophy (MSA) is a neurodegenerative syndrome that includes derangement of the extrapyramidal and pyramidal motor, autonomic, and cerebellar systems. The disorder can be subclassified for each patient on the basis of this pattern of involvement as MSA-parkinsonism (predominantly motor dysfunction), MSA-autonomic (predominantly autonomic type), and MSA-cerebellar (predominantly cerebellar type).[19] The prevalence of MSA is 4.4/100,000 people.[13] In a review of 203 patients with clinically diagnosed MSA, the male-to-female ratio was 1.3 to 1. Nearly half the patients presented with autonomic features, and almost all the others developed them over the course of the illness. Parkinsonism was usually symmetric. Although almost one third had tremor, a typical parkinsonian rest tremor was seen in <10%. Levodopa responsiveness was present in nearly one third of patients, but sustained benefits were present in only 13%. A subgroup of patients who responded well to levodopa had troublesome drug-induced midline involuntary movements and postures (ie, dystonic dyskinesias). Although cognitive impairment was common, severe dementia was rare.[20] Early diagnostic clues include early falling, autonomic dysfunction (ie, orthostatic hypotension, incontinence, impotence), absence of rest tremor, and failure to respond to levodopa.[21] Other signs include stridor, sleep apnea, involuntary gasping while awake, and prominent midline or facial involuntary movements precipitated by levodopa therapy.[20] Neuroimaging in MSA shows putaminal iron deposition, an intense rim on T2-weighted images at the lateral edge of the dorsolateral putamen or cruciform hyperintensivity in the pons ('hot cross bun sign').[22] MSA progresses more rapidly than PD. Nearly half the patients are markedly disabled or require a wheelchair within 5 years. Median survival is 9.5 years.[23]

Corticobasal degeneration

Corticobasal degeneration (CBD) was first reported in 1968. It is an exceptionally rare syndrome. The main features of this poorly understood neurodegenerative illness are parkinsonian and other movement disorders with apraxia, loss of cortical sensory functions, and myoclonus. In a review of 147 CBD patients seen at eight movement disorders centers, all had parkinsonian features and 89% had other movement disorders, including myoclonus, tremor, dystonia, and chorea.[24] Rigidity is prominent in the affected limbs. Apraxia is also prominent and disabling. In many patients, symptoms of alien limb develop.[25] Cortical sensory disturbances, such as extinction to double simultaneous stimulation and loss of 2-point discrimination and stereognosis, are common. The signs of CBD begin unilaterally, and profound asymmetry is characteristic. Cognitive function may be preserved, although 25% of patients with the classic syndrome have dementia.[24] The presentation of CBD varies quite a bit, and progressive aphasia, a PSP-like manifestation, or pure dementia may be seen.[26] Neuroimaging studies show prominent atrophy of the parietal lobe contralateral to the initially affected side.[22] Although about 25% of patients may have a favorable response to one or more therapeutic agents (including dopaminergic drugs and benzodiazepines), the outcome is generally disappointing.[24] The disease is inexorably progressive, leading to death from complications of immobility 6 to 8 years after onset.

Alzheimer's disease with extrapyramidal signs

AD is the most common degenerative dementia, responsible for >50% of dementia cases. The prevalence of AD increases exponentially with age, and the lifetime risk of AD is between 12% and 17%.[27] Typical AD begins with memory impairment, followed by deficits in other cortically based cognitive functions. Spontaneous extrapyramidal signs are common in AD, ranging in frequency from 12% to 30% of patients.[28,29] The frequency of parkinsonian signs seen in AD are in decreasing order—bradykinesia, gait disorder, rigidity, and tremor.[30] The presence or severity of parkinsonism in AD predicts a faster progression of the illness.[31] The parkinsonian signs in AD are not generally responsive to antiparkinsonian medications, which are poorly tolerated in this population. Another common problem in patients with AD is parkinsonism induced by neuroleptic drugs used to control behavior disturbances. In this population, the frequency of parkinsonian signs is 67%.[32]

Because AD and PD are common disorders, some patients will show clinical and pathologic evidence of both conditions. In these patients, extrapyramidal signs may be responsive to levodopa, but clinicians should watch for signs of increased confusion, hallucinations, or psychosis resulting from its use.

Diffuse Lewy body disease

Diffuse Lewy body disease (DLBD) is the second most common degenerative dementia, accounting for as many as 20% of dementia cases. The classic features of DLBD are fluctuating cognitive dysfunction, spontaneous parkinsonism, and hallucinations.[33] Patients with DLBD are extremely sensitive to antipsychotic medications, which can precipitate life-threatening parkinsonism.[34] Parkinsonism may be present at the outset or may develop after the dementia. Parkinsonism should not precede the dementia for more than 1 year. It is difficult to clinically diagnosis DLBD. A clinicopathologic study looking at interrater reliability of the diagnosis of DLBD from case vignettes showed a sensitivity of 28.6%.[35] The confusion stems from clinical overlap with PD, AD with extrapyramidal signs, and the Lewy body variant of AD.[34] There may be a response to dopaminergic therapy,[36] but caution must be exercised as these drugs invariably worsen the behavior syndrome.

Huntington's disease

Huntington's disease (HD) is an inherited, neurodegenerative disorder related to an expanded unstable trinucleotide (CAG) repeat in the IT15 or Huntington gene on chromosome 4. Onset is typically in the fourth or fifth decade with a motor disorder, and personality or affective disorder. The motor disorder may be complex, comprising choreic or dystonic involuntary movements combined with mild parkinsonian features. With disease advancement, slowness and gait disorder become more prominent and dementia supervenes. Parkinsonism and dystonia often dominate the end stage of the disorder. Although the inheritance pattern is autosomal dominant, a family history can be vague or shrouded in secrecy and new mutations from expansion of a borderline-length trinucleotide repeat have been well described. In some cases with large repeat expansions, the onset of the disorder is before age 21. The juvenile phenotype differs from the typical adult-onset phenotype in that parkinsonism and dystonia predominate from onset.[37] Because the parkinsonian phenotype almost exclusively occurs in early-onset HD, there is little overlap between HD and PD in the typical age range of PD onset. Neuroimaging studies often show atrophy of the caudate nucleus and putamen, but they are not reliable for diagnosis. A direct gene test is available.[38] No treatment exists for the degenerative process. Although parkinsonism in HD may improve with dopaminergic therapy, chorea and psychiatric disorders may worsen, so dopaminergic drugs are not routinely prescribed to treat HD.[39]

Wilson's disease

Wilson's disease (WD) was first completely described in 1912 by S.A.K. Wilson. The condition, which he called progressive lenticular degeneration, was characterized by involuntary movements, including a prominent bilateral tremor, slowness and spasticity of the limbs and face with a characteristic grimace (risus sardonicus), dysarthria and dysphagia, and emotional lability. Pathologically, the disease was typified by bilateral softening of the lenticular nuclei. WD is now known to be an extremely rare (prevalence 3/100,000 people) autosomal-recessive condition caused by one of several types of mutations localized to the ATP7B gene on chromosome 13. The disorder usually presents during the first two decades of life, although presentation up to age 58 has been reported.[40] Impaired biliary copper excretion leads to its deposition in the liver until storage is overwhelmed. Copper then accumulates in extrahepatic tissues, including the brain. WD may present with cirrhosis or fulminant hepatic failure, or a primary nervous system presentation. The mean age at presentation of the hepatic form is 11 years, and the mean age at presentation of the neurologic form is about 18 years. Tremor is often the presenting sign of central nervous system (CNS) disease. It may occur at rest and be indistinguishable from the tremor of parkinsonism or affect mainly posture and action. Decreased finger dexterity, rigidity, and decreased facial expression may also confuse the picture with parkinsonism. Progressive dysarthria with hypokinetic and spastic/ataxic qualities may lead to total anarthria. Chorea, dystonia, and a lurching gait are common. Psychiatric symptoms are also common, and include adjustment disorders, anxiety, depression, psychosis, and behavior disturbances. Systemic manifestations include renal disease, skeletal changes, and hemolytic anemia. Copper deposits in Descemet's membrane cause the characteristic Kayser-Fleischer ring, a golden brown ring around the limbus of the cornea. Although the rings are present in most patients with untreated WD, it may require a slit-lamp examination to detect them. Sunflower cataracts are rarely seen in WD. There is increased 24-hour excretion of copper. Magnetic resonance imaging (MRI) scans may show high signal lesions on T2-weighted images in the striatum, globus pallidus, thalamus, brainstem, or cerebellum along with cortical and subcortical atrophy.[40] WD is associated with low serum ceruloplasmin levels. Most clinicians diagnose WD when they find Kayser-Fleischer rings in the eyes, increased 24-hour urinary copper, and low serum ceruloplasmin. However, there are well-reported cases without Kayser-Fleischer rings at diagnosis.[40] The reliability of ceruloplasmin levels also has not been established. Ceruloplasmin is low in 20% of heterozygotes for the WD mutation, and about 5% of WD patients may have normal ceruloplasmin levels. Therefore, when suspicion for WD is high, clinicians must consider a liver biopsy to check for copper content. The disease is rapidly progressive and always fatal, if not treated. Treatments include D-penicillamine, trientine, tetrathiomolybdate (investigational), zinc supplementation, and copper restriction.[41]

Pantothenate-kinase-associated neurodegeneration

Pantothenate-kinase-associated neurodegeneration (PKAN) (formerly known as Hallervorden-Spatz disease) was described in 1922 as an autosomal-recessive disorder that causes dystonia, rigidity, choreoathetosis, dementia, and dysarthria associated with brown discoloration of the substantia nigra and globus pallidus. PKAN can be classified as classic, atypical, or intermediate. Classic PKAN presents between ages 7 and 12 with progressive rigidity, dysarthria, dysphagia, dystonia, and choreoathetoid movements, and is rapidly progressive to a nonambulatory state within 15 years. Mental deterioration and visual disturbance may occur. A pure akinetic-rigid syndrome has been reported. Atypical PKAN begins later and progresses more slowly. The intermediate classification includes late-onset rapidly progressive and early-onset slowly progressive forms of the illness. Late-onset disease has been confused with familial parkinsonism.[42] MRI brain scans may show iron deposits in the basal ganglia or the 'eye of the tiger' sign, a hyperintense region within the hypointense medial globus pallidus.[43] Various mutations have been described in the PARK2 gene on chromosome 20. Other causative mutations have been described in the phospholipase A2 group V (PLA2G5) gene on chromosome 22.[44] There is no known treatment, and the condition progresses to death in about 11 years.

Calcification of the basal ganglia

Many things cause calcium to deposit in the basal ganglia. Computed tomography (CT) scanning shows calcium deposits in the basal ganglia in up to 0.6% of people scanned. Other causes of calcium deposition in the basal ganglia are hypoparathyroidism, pseudohypoparathyroidism, hyperparathyroidism, and acquired brain injury (ie, anoxia at birth, carbon monoxide poisoning, lead poisoning, tuberous sclerosis, postinfectious inflammation, acquired immunodeficiency syndrome [AIDS], postradiation toxicity, mitochondrial encephalopathy, Down syndrome). Idiopathic calcification of the basal ganglia begins between ages 30 and 60. Progressive dysarthria, extrapyramidal signs, and ataxia are the salient clinical features of the illness. The disorder has been mapped to chromosome 14. There is no known treatment.

Creutzfeldt-Jakob disease

Creutzfeldt-Jakob disease (CJD) is a rare transmissible spongiform encephalopathy. It is caused by an abnormal configuration of the prion protein gene. Sporadic disease is believed to occur as the result of a posttranslational modification of the protein from the PrP(c) form. Sporadic CJD occurs with a frequency of 0.1/100,000 people. Onset of CJD averages at around 60 years. Men and women are affected in equal numbers. CJD presents with progressive cognitive impairment, nervousness, myoclonic and tremulous hand movements, and gait disorder. The electroencephalogram (EEG) may show slow, periodic complexes, often with a triphasic appearance. CJD can also be acquired from materials contaminated with the altered protein. Modes of infectious transmission include ingestion of infected brain tissue, corneal transplantation, inoculation of human growth hormone (hGH) and gonadotropin, infected depth electrodes, lyophilized dural grafts, and contaminated neurosurgical instruments.[45] Recently described cases of new-variant CJD have been linked to the ingestion of meat from cattle with 'mad cow' disease in Great Britain.[46] New-variant CJD presents at an earlier age (ie, around 30 years). Cognitive or behavior changes are the presenting signs. Myoclonus, choreoathetosis, an akinetic-rigid state, or tremor may be seen. EEG changes are typically not seen. All new-variant CJD cases have been found to be homozygous for the Met-129 polymorphism in the prion protein gene, suggesting genetic susceptibility to the disorder. The condition is rapidly progressive leading to death, usually within 2 years. About 15% of CJD cases are familial. Familial CJD is predominantly inherited and relates to mutations in the prion protein gene. Disease onset is usually earlier in familial cases than in sporadic cases. Gerstmann-Straussler disease and familial fatal insomnia variants are also related to prion protein gene mutations. Survival may be longer in familial compared with sporadic cases.

Acquired Structural Diseases and Parkinsonism

Subcortical vascular disease

Multiple subcortical infarctions, often associated with multi-infarct dementia, can cause a variety of gait disorders that may include features of parkinsonism. In a series of 25 such patients, all had parkinsonism, and most had either ataxia or apraxia or both.[47] Several clinical parkinsonian syndromes may be seen in the context of vascular disease. There are also patients who meet the clinical criteria for PD, and these cases may relate to coincident PD in the context of vascular disease. In other cases, unilateral parkinsonism begins in the setting of an acute ischemic or hemorrhagic stroke. Finally, vascular parkinsonism may present as an atypical parkinsonism with predominant involvement of the lower body and poor response to levodopa. Rest tremor is usually absent. Examination may also show focal pyramidal tract signs, dementia, pseudobulbar palsy, or dementia.[48] Typical neuroimaging changes are ventricular enlargement, leukoariosis, and vermian atrophy.[47]

Hydrocephalus

Both communicating and noncommunicating hydrocephalus have been reported to cause parkinsonism.[49] Obstructive hydrocephalus caused by aqueductal stenosis or tumor has been reported to cause levodopa-responsive parkinsonism that usually improves after shunting.[50] Normal pressure hydrocephalus, a controversial entity in which the cerebral ventricles are enlarged without an increase in cerebrospinal fluid (CSF) pressure, is commonly associated with gait disorder with cognitive dysfunction and urinary incontinence. Virtually all parkinsonian signs have been described in hydrocephalus patients, and some are responsive to levodopa.[51] In carefully selected patients, surgical ventricular drainage may lead to improvements in cognition, gait, and bladder function. A recent study of long-term outcome following CSF shunting procedures suggests that it is more effective for motor than cognitive function at 5 years, and that patients <75 years at the time of surgery and those with better preoperative function fared better than others.[52]

Brain tumor

Parkinsonism is a rare manifestation of brain tumor. It has been reported with craniopharyngioma, sphenoid ridge, or frontal convexity meningioma.[53,54] Atypical features, such as visual field abnormality or pyramidal motor deficits, help distinguish a brain tumor from PD. Histopathologic examination shows damage to the substantia nigra, striatum, or both.[54] If presynaptic dopamine loss exists, the symptoms may be partially amenable to dopaminergic therapy.

Subdural hematoma

Subdural hematoma that causes or exacerbates parkinsonism has been reported.[55] Patients with subdural hematoma can present with parkinsonism,[56] or the disorder can worsen pre-existing, drug-induced parkinsonism (DIP) or parkinsonism of other etiologies.[55] Clues to this diagnosis include a subacute evolution of parkinsonian signs, and coexisting lethargy or cognitive dysfunction. Parkinsonism in these cases has been reported to improve or resolve following surgical drainage of the hematoma.[55]

Anoxic brain injury

A few reports associate parkinsonism with hypoxic brain injury. In one case, neuroimaging studies showed low-density lesions in the putamina.[57] In such cases, the diagnosis is obvious and not confused with PD. Do not expect a positive response to dopaminergic therapy.

Traumatic brain injury

A rapidly progressive akinetic-rigid syndrome has been reported to follow severe closed head injury.[58] Parkinsonian signs are frequently seen in the dementia pugilistica syndrome that follows repeated head injury as seen in boxers. The syndrome includes all the cardinal signs of parkinsonism, usually accompanied by cerebellar or pyramidal signs, as well as dysarthria and mental status changes.[59] Pathologic changes in pugilistic parkinsonism include loss of cells in the substantia nigra without Lewy bodies.[60] Although some epidemiologic evidence shows that head injury is a risk factor for PD, no supporting evidence exists that minor head injury causes the acute or subacute development of PD.[61]

Toxic brain injury

Reports show several neurotoxic agents cause parkinsonism. The most important is 1-methyl-4-phenyl-1,2,3,6-tetrahydropyridine (MPTP), an inadvertent contaminant of a meperidine analogue designer drug. It caused acute severe parkinsonism in several drug addicts in California.[62] A chemist working with MPTP also developed parkinsonism. Although this condition affects only a few people and ongoing exposure is not an issue, the compound has proved invaluable in the study of PD. Clinicians use MPTP in rodent and primate models to simulate PD.

Carbon monoxide

Acute, severe carbon monoxide poisoning is frequently associated with coma. Survivors can have neurologic sequelae including personality or behavior changes, confusion, memory, and visuospatial abnormalities. Pure parkinsonism or a state of akinetic-mutism can develop. Sequelae follows a progressive course, or the patient may improve and then suffer a relapse.[63] A variable response of parkinsonian signs to antiparkinsonian therapy has been reported.[64,65]

Manganese

Manganism was first reported in 1837. Manganese exposure usually occurs by inhalation. Occupational exposure occurs during manganese mining and in ferromanganese factories. Arc welders may also be at risk. Headaches, asthenia, somnolence, and social withdrawal are early signs, and personality changes are common. Parkinsonism usually develops. Speech may be severely affected, and the patient may experience coarse tremor and dystonia. Symptoms can progress long after exposure ends. Do not use blood and urinary manganese levels to make a diagnosis.[66] Neuroimaging abnormalities include areas of increased signal on T1-weighted images in the globus pallidus, striatum, and midbrain.[67] In well-documented cases, PET scans do not show a presynaptic dopamine deficit, clearly distinguishing the disorder from PD.[67] The reported response to antidopaminergic agents varies,[68] although most authors report no benefit.[67,68]

Clinicians have recently attempted to link manganese exposure, particularly occupational exposure in welders, to the subsequent development of PD. However, published studies show significant methodologic weaknesses, and no definitive link has been established.[69]

Cyanide

Several reports exist of parkinsonian signs in patients who have survived accidental or intentional cyanide ingestion. Dystonic signs are a common accompaniment. Neuroimaging studies show lesions in the putamen and globus pallidus bilaterally.[70]

Carbon disulfide

Carbon disulfide poisoning is associated with irritability, cognitive decline, psychiatric symptoms, delirium, parkinsonism, and peripheral neuropathy. An epidemiologic study suggested occupational exposure to carbon disulfide might predispose people to develop parkinsonism.[71]

Methanol

Methanol intoxication has been linked to several neurologic symptoms including parkinsonism, pyramidal signs, and dementia. Lesions of the white matter and putamen have been described,[72] and the response to antiparkinsonian therapy varies.[72,73]

Drug-induced Parkinsonism

In a review of parkinsonian disorders in the Olmsted County, Minnesota study, 20% of parkinsonism patients were found to have DIP. Dopamine receptor blocking agents, such as neuroleptics or antiemetics, are usually implicated.[74,75] Older women and those treated with higher-potency agents are most at risk. The calcium-channel antagonists cinnarizine and flunarizine, which are not available in the United States, have been linked to the development of DIP. The role of other calcium-channel antagonists in parkinsonism is unknown.[76] Recovery can take as long as 6 months once the offending drug is discontinued. In some patients with significant disability, treatment with amantadine (Symmetrel®) or carbidopa/levodopa (Sinemet®, Sinemet® CR) may be required.

Practical Approach to the Diagnosis of Parkinsonism

Clinicians who suspect a patient has parkinsonism must take a detailed history, including disease onset and progression, precipitating factors, family history, drug exposures within the previous 6 months before onset, and other medical conditions. The physical examination should focus on identifying the cardinal signs of parkinsonism as well as atypical features that might suggest alternate diagnoses (Tables 2-2 and 2-3). Laboratory studies should include thyroid function tests to exclude hypothyroidism. A neuroimaging study, preferably a MRI, is usually recommended. Clinical neurophysiology studies, such as an EEG, evoked potentials, and an EMG, are of no clinical use. Recognizing that atypical symptoms and signs may evolve during the illness, clinicians should devote continued attention to patient history and physical examination. Moreover, unexpected developments, such as unresponsiveness to medical therapy or the appearance of unusual symptoms, should prompt a reassessment of the diagnosis.

References

1. Meara J, Bhowmick BK, Hobson P: Accuracy of diagnosis in patients with presumed Parkinson's disease. *Age Ageing* 1999;28:99-102.

2. Jellinger K: The pathology of parkinsonism. In: Marsden CD, Fahn S, eds: *Movement Disorders*, 2nd ed. London, England, Butterworths, 1987, pp 124-167.

3. Shih MC, Hoexter MQ, et al: Parkinson's disease and dopamine transporter neuroimaging: a critical review. *Sao Paulo Med J* 2006;124:168-175.

4. Hughes AJ, Ben-Shlomo Y, Daniel SE, et al: What features improve the accuracy of clinical diagnosis in Parkinson's disease: a clinicopathologic study. *Neurology* 1992;42:1142-1146; erratum *Neurology* 1992;42:1436.

5. Brooks DJ: The early diagnosis of Parkinson's disease. *Ann Neurol* 1998;44:S10-S18.

6. Lees AJ: When did Ray Kennedy's Parkinson's disease begin? *Mov Disord* 1992;7:110-116.

7. Abbott RD, Petrovitch H, White LR, et al: Frequency of bowel movements and the future risk of Parkinson's disease. *Neurology* 2001;57:456-462.

8. Leentjens AF, Van den Akker M, Metsemakers JF, et al: Higher incidence of depression preceding the onset of Parkinson's disease: a register study. *Mov Disord* 2003;18:414-418.

9. Hely MA, Morris JG, Reid WG, et al: Sydney Multicenter Study of Parkinson's disease: non-L-dopa-responsive problems dominate at 15 years. *Mov Disord* 2005;20:190-199.

10. Poewe WH, Wenning GK: The natural history of Parkinson's disease. *Neurology* 1996;47:S146-S152.

11. Stern PH, McDowell F, Miller JM, et al: Levodopa therapy effects on natural history of Parkinsonism. *Arch Neurol* 1972;27:481-485.

12. Hoehn MM, Yahr MD: Parkinsonism: onset, progression and mortality. *Neurology* 1967;17:427-442.

13. Schrag A, Ben-Shlomo Y, Quinn NP: Prevalence of progressive supranuclear palsy and multiple system atrophy: a cross-sectional study. *Lancet* 1999;354:1771-1775.

14. de Yebenes JG, Sarasa JL, Daniel SE, et al: Familial progressive supranuclear palsy. Description of a pedigree and review of the literature. *Brain* 1995;118:1095-1103.

15. Litvan I, Grimes DA, Lang AE, et al: Clinical features differentiating patients with postmortem confirmed progressive supranuclear palsy and corticobasal degeneration. *J Neurol* 1999;246(suppl 2): II1-II5.

16. Barsottini OG, Ferraz HB, Maia AC Jr, et al: Differentiation of Parkinson's disease and progressive supranuclear palsy with magnetic resonance imaging: The first Brazilian experience. *Parkinsonism Relat Disord* 2007; Epub ahead of publication.

17. Kompoliti K, Goetz CG, Litvan I, et al: Pharmacological therapy in progressive supranuclear palsy. *Arch Neurol* 1998;55: 1099-1102.

18. Golbe LI, Davis PH, Schoenberg BS, et al: Prevalence and natural history of progressive supranuclear palsy. *Neurology* 1988;38:1031-1034.

19. Austin MT, Davis TL, Robertson D, et al: Multiple system atrophy: clinical presentation and diagnosis. *Tenn Med* 1999;92:55-57.

20. Wenning GK, Tison F, Ben Shlomo Y, et al: Multiple system atrophy: a review of 203 pathologically proven cases. *Mov Disord* 1997;12:133-147.

21. Fearnley JM, Lees AJ: Striatonigral degeneration. A clinicopathological study. *Brain* 1990;113:1823-1842.

22. Arai K: MRI of progressive supranuclear palsy, corticobasal degeneration and multiple system atrophy. *J Neurol* 2006;253(suppl 3):iii25-iii29.

23. Wenning GK, Ben Shlomo Y, Magalhaes M, et al: Clinical features and natural history of multiple system atrophy. An analysis of 100 cases. *Brain* 1994;117:835-845.

24. Kompoliti K, Goetz CG, Boeve BF, et al: Clinical presentation and pharmacological therapy in corticobasal degeneration. *Arch Neurol* 1998;55:957-961.

25. Riley DE, Lang AE: Corticobasal ganglionic degeneration (CBGD): further observations in six additional cases. *Neurology* 1988;38(suppl 1):360.

26. Bergeron C, Davis A, Lang AE: Corticobasal ganglionic degeneration and progressive supranuclear palsy presenting with cognitive decline. *Brain Pathol* 1998;8:355-365.

27. Rocca WA, Cha RH, Waring SC, et al: Incidence of dementia and Alzheimer's disease: a reanalysis of data from Rochester, Minnesota, 1975-1984. *Am J Epidemiol* 1998;148:51-62.

28. Burns A, Jacoby R, Levy R: Neurological signs in Alzheimer's disease. *Age Ageing* 1991;20:45-51.

29. Mitchell SL: Extrapyramidal features in Alzheimer's disease. *Age Ageing* 1999;28:401-409.

30. Lopez OL, Wisnieski SR, Becker JT, et al: Extrapyramidal signs in patients with probable Alzheimer disease. *Arch Neurol* 1997;54:969-975.

31. Chui HC, Lyness SA, Sobel E, et al: Extrapyramidal signs and psychiatric symptoms predict faster cognitive decline in Alzheimer's disease. *Arch Neurol* 1994;51:676-681.

32. Caligiuri MP, Rockwell E, Jeste DV: Extrapyramidal side effects in patients with Alzheimer's disease treated with low-dose neuroleptic medication. *Am J Geriatr Psychiatry* 1998;6:75-82.

33. Benecke R: Diffuse Lewy body disease—a clinical syndrome or a disease entity? *J Neurol* 2003;250(suppl 1):I39-I42.

34. Hohl U, Tiraboschi P, Hansen LA, et al: Diagnostic accuracy of dementia with Lewy bodies. *Arch Neurol* 2000;57:347-351.

35. Litvan I, MacIntyre A, Goetz CG, et al: Accuracy of the clinical diagnoses of Lewy body disease, Parkinson disease, and dementia with Lewy bodies: a clinicopathologic study. *Arch Neurol* 1998;55:969-978.

36. Louis ED, Goldman JE, Powers JM, et al: Parkinsonian features of eight pathologically diagnosed cases of diffuse Lewy body disease. *Mov Disord* 1995;10:188-194.

37. van Dijk JG, van der Velde EA, Roos RA, et al: Juvenile Huntington disease. *Hum Genet* 1986;73:235-239.

38. A novel gene containing a trinucleotide repeat that is expanded and unstable on Huntington's disease chromosomes. The Huntington's Disease Collaborative Research Group. *Cell* 1993;72:971-983.

39. Tan BK, Leijnse-Ybema HJ, Brand HJ: Levodopa in Huntington's chorea. *Lancet* 1972;1:903.

40. Ala A, Walker AP, Ashkan A, et al: Wilson's disease. *Lancet* 2007;369:397-408.

41. Brewer GJ, Yuzbasiyan-Gurkan V: Wilson disease. *Medicine (Baltimore)* 1992;71:139-164.

42. Jankovic J, Kirkpatrick JB, Blomquist KA, et al: Late-onset Hallervorden-Spatz disease presenting as familial parkinsonism. *Neurology* 1985;35:227-234.

43. Angelini L, Nardocci N, Rumi V, et al: Hallervorden-Spatz disease: clinical and MRI study of 11 cases diagnosed in life. *J Neurol* 1992;239:417-425.

44. Hayflick SJ: Neurodegeneration with brain iron accumulation: from genes to pathogenesis. *Semin Pediatr Neurol* 2006;13:182-185.

45. Alter M: How is Creutzfeldt-Jakob disease acquired? *Neuroepidemiology* 2000;19:55-61.

46. Gordon N: New variant Creutzfeldt-Jakob disease. *Int J Clin Pract* 1999;53:456-459.

47. Thajeb P: Gait disorders of multi-infarct dementia. CT and clinical correlation. *Acta Neurol Scand* 1993;87:239-242.

48. Rektor I, Rektorova I, Kubova D: Vascular parkinsonism—an update. *J Neurol Sci* 2006;248:185-191.

49. Murrow RW, Schweiger GD, Kepes JJ, et al: Parkinsonism due to a basal ganglia lacunar state: clinicopathologic correlation. *Neurology* 1990;40:897-900.

50. Curran T, Lang AE: Parkinsonian syndromes associated with hydrocephalus: case reports, a review of the literature, and pathophysiological hypotheses. *Mov Disord* 1994;9:508-520.

51. Clough CG: A case of normal pressure hydrocephalus presenting as levodopa responsive parkinsonism. *J Neurol Neurosurg Psychiatry* 1987;50:234.

52. Kahlon B, Sjunnesson J, et al: Long-term outcome in patients with suspected normal pressure hydrocephalus. *Neurosurgery* 2007; 60:327-332; discussion 332.

53. Kondo T: (Brain tumor and parkinsonism). *Nippon Rinsho* 1997; 55:118-122.

54. Garcia de Yebenes J, Gervas JJ, Iglesias J, et al: Biochemical findings in a case of parkinsonism secondary to brain tumor. *Ann Neurol* 1982;11:313-316.

55. Wiest RG, Burgunder JM, Krauss JK: Chronic subdural haematomas and Parkinsonian syndromes. *Acta Neurochir (Wien)* 1999;141:753-757; discussion 757-758.

56. Krul JM, Wokke JH: Bilateral subdural hematoma presenting as subacute parkinsonism. *Clin Neurol Neurosurg* 1987;89:107-109.

57. Matsuda M, Kondo K, Yanagisawa N: (A case of parkinsonism after resuscitation from cardiac arrest showing low density areas in the bilateral putamen with computed tomography). *Rinsho Shinkeigaku* 1987;27:325-328.

58. Bhatt M, Desai J, Mankodi A, et al: Posttraumatic akinetic-rigid syndrome resembling Parkinson's disease: a report on three patients. *Mov Disord* 2000;15:313-317.

59. Critchley M: Medical aspects of boxing, particularly from a neurologic standpoint. *Br Med J* 1957;1:357-362.

60. Johnson J: Organic psychosyndromes due to boxing. *Br J Psychiatry* 1969;115:45-53.

61. Factor SA, Sanchez-Ramos J, Weiner WJ: Trauma as an etiology of parkinsonism: a historical review of the concept. *Mov Disord* 1988;3:30-36.

62. Langston JW, Ballard P: Parkinsonism induced by 1-methyl-4-phenyl-1,2,3,6-tetrahydropyridine (MPTP): implications for treatment and the pathogenesis of Parkinson's disease. *Can J Neurol Sci* 1984;11:160-165.

63. Lee MS, Marsden CD: Neurological sequelae following carbon monoxide poisoning clinical course and outcome according to the clinical types and brain computed tomography scan findings. *Mov Disord* 1994;9:550-558.

64. Klawans HL, Stein RW, Tanner CM, et al: A pure parkinsonian syndrome following acute carbon monoxide intoxication. *Arch Neurol* 1982;39:302-304.

65. Tack E, de Reuck J: The use of bromocriptine in parkinsonism after carbon monoxide poisoning. *Clin Neurol Neurosurg* 1987;89:275-279.

66. Apostoli P, Lucchini R, Alessio L: Are current biomarkers suitable for the assessment of manganese exposure in individual workers? *Am J Ind Med* 2000;37:283-290.

67. Pal PK, Samii A, Calne DB: Manganese neurotoxicity: a review of clinical features, imaging and pathology. *Neurotoxicology* 1999;20:227-238.

68. Huang CC, Lu CS, Chu NS, et al: Progression after chronic manganese exposure. *Neurology* 1993;43:1479-1483.

69. Jankovic J: Searching for a relationship between manganese and welding and Parkinson's disease. *Neurology* 2005;64:2021-2028.

70. Rosenberg NL, Myers JA, Martin WR: Cyanide-induced parkinsonism: clinical, MRI, and 6-fluorodopa PET studies. *Neurology* 1989;39:142-144.

71. Ohlson CG, Hogstedt C: Parkinson's disease and occupational exposure to organic solvents, agricultural chemicals and mercury— a case-referent study. *Scand J Work Environ Health* 1981;7:252-256.

72. McLean DR, Jacobs H, Mielke BW: Methanol poisoning: a clinical and pathological study. *Ann Neurol* 1980;8:161-167.

73. Davis LE, Adair JC: Parkinsonism from methanol poisoning: benefit from treatment with anti-Parkinson drugs. *Mov Disord* 1999;14:520-522.

74. Tison F, Lecaroz J, Letenneur L, et al: Parkinsonism and exposure to neuroleptic drugs in elderly people living in institutions. *Clin Neuropharmacol* 1999;22:5-10.

75. Miller LG, Jankovic J: Metoclopramide-induced movement disorders. Clinical findings with a review of the literature. *Arch Intern Med* 1989;149:2486-2492.

76. Garcia-Ruiz PJ, Garcia de Yebenes J, Jimenez-Jimenez FJ, et al: Parkinsonism associated with calcium channel blockers: a prospective follow-up study. *Clin Neuropharmacol* 1992;15:19-26.

2

Chapter 3

Pathology, Pathophysiology, and Pathogenesis

Pathology

In 1817, James Parkinson concluded that the pathology site in 'shaking palsy' was the medulla spinalis, extending with disease progression to the medulla oblongata.[1] The first pathology description in the substantia nigra in Parkinson's disease (PD) is attributed to Trétiakoff (1919).[2] However, the importance of the Lewy body, first described in the substantia innominata by Lewy in 1913, to PD was not known until years later.

The typical pathologic changes of PD are neuronal loss with gliosis and cytoplasmic inclusions (ie, Lewy bodies), which are smooth, rounded inclusions with an eosinophilic core and pale halo. Lewy bodies are found in conditions other than PD, including in patients diagnosed with neurologic illness, but are common in the primary Lewy body illnesses, PD, and diffuse Lewy body disease (DLBD).[3] Lewy bodies stain positively for ubiquitin and α-synuclein.[4] Recent clinicopathologic studies suggest that the earliest central nervous system (CNS) changes are seen in the anterior olfactory nucleus and in the dorsal motor nucleus of the glossopharyngeal and vagal nerves in the medulla oblongata. The changes ascend through the pons and into the midbrain, where they particularly affect dopaminergic neurons of the substantia nigra pars compacta (SNpc). These changes in the substantia nigra are associated with the typical cardinal motor disease signs. Later, there is progressive involvement of the cerebral cortex. This new evidence helps to explain early signs of PD that had for many years been thought to be risk factors, such as personality changes, affective and autonomic changes, as well as the evolution of symptoms in late-stage disease that do not respond to dopaminergic therapy.[5] Lewy bodies and degenerative changes are also found in the spinal cord, sympathetic ganglia, and myenteric plexus.

Researchers estimate that the cardinal motor symptoms of PD first appear after 50% to 80% of dopaminergic neurons in the SNpc have been lost,[6] resulting in a decrease of dopamine in the striatum, the projection site for neurons in the SNpc. Although the motor signs of PD are overwhelmingly related to dopamine deficiency, other signs and symptoms of PD relate to other known neurochemical changes. For example, autonomic changes may relate to reduced epinephrine and norepinephrine, affective changes may relate to serotonin or norepinephrine deficiencies, and cognitive changes may relate to acetylcholine (ACh) deficiency.

Pathophysiology

The basal ganglia include four nuclei—the striatum (composed of the caudate and putamen), the globus pallidus (composed of the internal and external segments), the subthalamic nucleus, and the substantia nigra. Five parallel loops (the motor, oculomotor, dorsolateral prefrontal, lateral orbitofrontal, and limbic) negotiate the cortico-striato-pallido-thalamo-cortical relay pathway, each with both a direct and an indirect pathway. Although movement disorder studies seem to focus on the motor pathway, all five parallel loops are important in understanding these conditions.

The basal ganglia motor function model was developed in the 1980s and is shown in Figure 3-1. Afferent inputs from the cerebral cortex converge on the putamen, from which two pathways arise. The direct pathway inhibitory

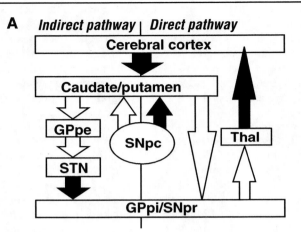

Figure 3-1: Model of basal ganglia function in (A) normal state, (B) parkinsonism, and (C) chorea. The relative activities of the direct and indirect pathways influence the initiation, speed, and purity of movement. The direct pathway, which facilitates thalamocortical activity, helps with movement, initiation, and maintenance. This pathway is facilitated by dopamine. The indirect pathway inhibits thalamocortical activity and is important in braking movement and preventing the intrusion of unwanted movement. This pathway is inhibited by dopamine. In parkinsonism (B), loss of dopaminergic activity reduces activity in the direct pathway and increases activity in the indirect pathway, thereby reducing thalamocortical activity that leads to paucity and reduced amplitude of movement. Neuronal activity in the subthalamic nucleus and globus pallidus is pathologically increased in parkinsonism, which explains the benefits of ablative surgery performed in these targets. In chorea (C), excess dopaminergic activity leads to increased activity in the direct pathway and reduced activity in the indirect pathway. Neuronal firing is reduced in the subthalamic nucleus and globus pallidus pars interna.

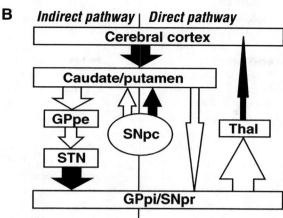

B

Indirect pathway | Direct pathway

Cerebral cortex

Caudate/putamen

GPpe

SNpc

STN

Thal

GPpi/SNpr

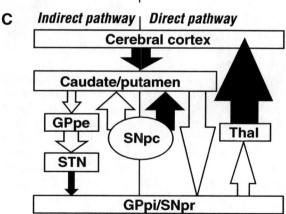

C

Indirect pathway | Direct pathway

Cerebral cortex

Caudate/putamen

GPpe

SNpc

STN

Thal

GPpi/SNpr

GPpe=globus pallidus pars externa, GPpi=globus pallidus pars interna, SNpc=substantia nigra pars compacta, SNpr=substantia nigra pars reticulata, STN=subthalamic nucleus, Thal=thalamus. Filled arrows indicate excitatory activity; open arrows indicate inhibitory activity.

efferents synapse on neurons in the globus pallidus pars interna (GPpi) and its homologous structure, the substantia nigra pars reticulata (SNpr), from which inhibitory efferents travel to the thalamus. Excitatory thalamocortical efferents return to the cerebral cortex. Activity in the direct pathway facilitates cortical activity.

Indirect pathway inhibitory efferents synapse on the neurons of the globus pallidus externa (GPpe), from which inhibitory efferents synapse on the subthalamic nucleus. Excitatory efferents arising from the subthalamic nucleus travel to the GPpi, from which inhibitory efferents synapse in the thalamus on the neurons that give rise to thalamo-cortical pathways. Activity in the indirect pathway inhibits cortical activity. The direct and indirect pathways have opposite actions on the GPpi. Activity in the direct pathway inhibits activity, while activity in the indirect pathway facilitates activity in the GPpi. Since the GPpi inhibits the thalamus, activity in the direct pathway facilitates thalamo-cortical activity, while activity in the indirect pathway inhibits thalamocortical activity.

In simple terms, the direct pathway facilitates activity in cortical motor pathways, and the indirect pathway inhibits activity in cortical motor pathways. Therefore, the direct pathway initiates and maintains motor activity and the indirect pathway focuses movement, including suppressing extraneous or involuntary movements.[7] The putamen also receives important afferent input from the SNpc. This dopaminergic pathway facilitates activity in the direct pathway and inhibits activity in the indirect pathway. Thus, dopamine deficiency causes direct pathway underactivity and indirect pathway overactivity, decreasing movement (as in PD). Dopamine excess (as in levdopa-treated advanced PD) causes direct pathway overactivity and indirect pathway underactivity, thereby causing involuntary movements, such as chorea or athetosis. Data from positron emission tomography (PET) scan images and from direct microelectrode recording of neuronal firing in the globus pallidus and subthalamic nucleus support the notion that in PD, direct pathway activity is reduced and indirect pathway activity is increased, leading to overactivity of the subthalamic nucleus and GPpi and suppression of cortical activity.[8] Similar evidence in patients with levodopa-induced chorea suggests that direct pathway activity is increased and indirect pathway activity is reduced, leading to underactivity of the subthalamic nucleus and GPpe and excessive cortical activity.[9]

The explosion in surgical treatment of advanced PD results from increased understanding of this pathophysiology. Surgical ablation of the overly active GPpi reduces bradykinesia, rigidity, and tremor contralateral to the operated side, as does high-frequency, low-amplitude electrical stimulation delivered to the nucleus by an implanted electrical stimulator. High-frequency, low-amplitude stimulation of the overactive subthalamic nucleus has become the preferred surgical approach (see Chapter 7).

Pathogenesis

The pathogenesis of PD remains unknown. However, insights have been provided by the discovery of genes responsible for hereditary parkinsonism. The discovery that dominantly inherited parkinsonism can result from mutation, duplication, or triplication of α-synuclein genes pointed to a pivotal role of this protein in PD-associated neurodegeneration. α-Synuclein is a protein of unknown function associated with the synaptic vesicle, which makes up a significant component of the Lewy body core.[10] Researchers have theorized that the mutant protein assumes an abnormal conformation, causing various intracellular derangements and producing aggregates that overwhelm the cell's housekeeping functions.[11] Autosomal-recessive, early-onset parkinsonism that is associated with the parkin, phosphatase, and tensin homolog (PTEN)-induced putative kinase 1 (PINK1), and DJ-1 (PARK7) genes appear to relate to derangements in mitochondrial function or to reduced resistance to oxidative stress. A small number of parkinsonism cases occurred after the recreational use of a meperidine analogue, which was contaminated with the mitochondrial protoxin 1-methyl-4-phenyl-1,2,3,6-tetra-hydropyridine (MPTP),[12] a pure environmental form of parkinsonism. Other environmental risk factors thought to be important in sporadic PD include head injury and exposure to pesticides or other toxic chemicals. These genetic and environmental findings suggest that the pathogenesis of PD relates strongly to mitochondrial impairment, oxidative stress, and disordered intracellular protein homeostasis.[13] Further genetic and environmental studies will increase our understanding of PD pathogenesis and will aid in the search for effective therapies.

References

1.   Parkinson J: *An Essay On the Shaking Palsy.* London, England, Whittingham and Rowland, 1817.

2.   Trétiakoff C: *Contribution a l'Etude de l'Anatomie du Locus Niger.* Paris, France, These de Paris, 1919.

3.   Uitti RJ, Calne DB: Pathogenesis of idiopathic parkinsonism. *Eur Neurol* 1993;33(suppl 1):6-23.

4.   Johnson WG: Late-onset neurodegenerative diseases—the role of protein insolubility. *J Anat* 2000;196:609-616.

5.   Braak H, Del Tredici K, Rub U, et al: Staging of brain pathology related to sporadic Parkinson's disease. *Neurobiol Aging* 2003;24:197-211.

6.   Jellinger K: The pathology of parkinsonism. In: Marsden CD, Fahn S, eds: *Movement Disorders,* 2nd ed. London, England, Butterworths, 1987, pp 124-167.

7.   Alexander GE, Crutcher MD: Functional architecture of basal ganglia circuits: neural substrates of parallel processing. *Trends Neurosci* 1990;13:266-271.

8.   Vitek JL, Bakay RA, Hashimoto T, et al: Microelectrode-guided pallidotomy: technical approach and its application in medically intractable Parkinson's disease. *J Neurosurg* 1998;88:1027-1043.

9.   Papa SM, Desimone R, Fiorani M, et al: Internal globus pallidus discharge is nearly suppressed during levodopa-induced dyskinesias. *Ann Neurol* 1999;46:732-738.

10. Spillantini MG, Crowther RA, Jakes R, et al: α-Synuclein in filamentous inclusions of Lewy bodies from Parkinson's disease and dementia with Lewy bodies. *Proc Natl Acad Sci USA* 1998;95: 6469-6473.

11. Golbe LI: α-Synuclein and Parkinson's disease. *Mov Disord* 1999;14:6-9.

12. Langston JW, Ballard P: Parkinsonism induced by 1-methyl-4-phenyl-1,2,3,6-tetrahydropyridine (MPTP): implications for treatment and the pathogenesis of Parkinson's disease. *Can J Neurol Sci* 1984;11:160-165.

13. Eriksen JL, Wszolek Z, Petrucelli L: Molecular pathogenesis of Parkinson disease. *Arch Neurol* 2005;62:353-357.

3

Chapter 4

Pharmacology of Parkinson's Disease

The concept that brain chemistry might prove important in the study of neurologic disease first emerged in the late 19th century, but was incompletely studied at that time.[1] The first suggestion that the substantia nigra was important in Parkinson's disease (PD) came in 1919, when lesions in this structure were found in patients with PD and postencephalitic parkinsonism.[2] For many years, dopamine was considered little more than an intermediary product in the biosynthesis of norepinephrine. However, in the late 1950s, researchers discovered that dopamine had a regional distribution in the brain that was different from that of norepinephrine. Moreover, similarities were found between the symptoms of reserpine-induced motor dysfunction and PD, suggesting a role for dopamine in parkinsonism. Finally, in the 1960s, the link was established between dopamine depletion in the substantia nigra and PD. Specific pharmacotherapy with high-dose levodopa followed in the late 1960s. Investigators believe that symptoms of PD first become apparent when 50% to 80% of substantia nigra neurons have degenerated, resulting in a loss of dopaminergic activity in the striatal targets of these neurons. More recent study has identified a number of other primary and secondary neurochemical changes that are important in PD.

Dopamine

Additional study has identified eight dopaminergic projection systems in the brain, two of which (mesostriatal and mesolimbocortical) arise from the ventral mesencephalon. In the 1970s, two types of dopamine receptors were differentiated, D_1-like receptors, which are linked to adenylate cyclase, and D_2-like receptors. Gene cloning in the 1980s further classified dopamine receptors into two families and five subtypes. The D_1-like family of dopamine receptors includes D_1 and D_5 receptors, and the D_2-like family of dopamine receptors includes D_2, D_3, and D_4 receptors.[3]

D_1-like receptors are found in the basal ganglia, where they function prominently in the direct pathway. Dopaminergic neurons that are destined to synapse on D_1-like receptors co-localize γ-aminobutyric acid (GABA), substance P, and dynorphin. D_1-like receptors are also found in the cerebral cortex and in the limbic system.

D_2-like receptors are found in the indirect pathway of the striatum, as well as in the cerebral cortex, limbic system, and pituitary gland. Neurons synapsing on D_2-like receptors in the indirect pathway co-localize GABA and enkephalin. These differences in co-localized substances allow identification of dopamine receptor subtypes in postmortem tissue. Through positron emission tomography (PET) and single-photon emission computed tomography (SPECT),[4] radiopharmaceutical agents that selectively label these populations of receptors are proving useful in the study of PD pharmacology in living patients.

Dopamine is synthesized within neuronal terminals from the precursor tyrosine by the sequential actions of tyrosine hydroxylase (rate-limiting enzyme) and L-aromatic acid decarboxylase. Dopamine is transported into storage vesicles by a transporter protein. Release is triggered by depolarization and entry of calcium and allows dopamine to act at postsynaptic receptors. Dopamine is metabolized by catechol-o-methyltransferase (COMT) and monoamine oxidase (MAO) (Figure 4-1).

In dopamine deficiency states, central levels of dopamine can be increased by the administration of its precursor, levodopa. Levodopa undergoes extensive metabolism

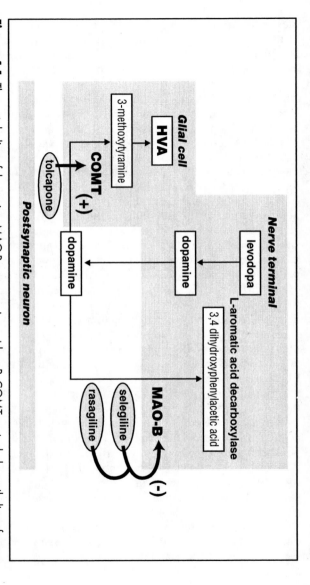

Figure 4-1: The metabolism of dopamine. MAO-B=monoamine oxidase B; COMT=catechol-o-methyltransferase; HVA=homovanillic acid.

outside of the central nervous system (CNS), and only a small fraction appears to cross the blood-brain barrier. For this reason, levodopa is nearly always administered in a combination tablet with a peripherally acting inhibitor of L-aromatic amino acid decarboxylase (carbidopa or benserazide), allowing increased CNS penetration. MAO inhibition with the selective monoamine oxidase B (MAO-B) inhibitors selegiline (Eldepryl®, Zelapar®) and rasagiline (Azilect®) appears to prolong the central pharmacologic effect of a dose of levodopa by reducing its degradation by MAO.

In the past several years, drugs have become available that block peripheral (entacapone [COMTan®]) or both peripheral and central (tolcapone [Tasmar®]) COMT activity, and increase the penetration of a drug into the CNS or prolong its pharmacologic activity at the dopamine receptor.

A number of direct-acting dopamine agonists are available. The two major classes of agents are the ergot-derived, such as bromocriptine (Parlodel®, Parlodel® SnapTabs®) and pergolide (Permax®), and the nonergot agonists, ie, pramipexole (Mirapex®) and ropinirole (Requip®). Pergolide was voluntarily withdrawn from the market and is no longer available in the United States, although it is available elsewhere. A nonergot dopamine agonist (ie, rotigotine) for transdermal delivery (Neupro® transdermal patch) was recently approved.[5] Dopamine agonists also differ in half-life and profile of receptor-subtype stimulation.[6]

Antidopaminergic drugs important in the treatment of PD include the typical and atypical neuroleptics. Typical neuroleptics include phenothiazines, such as chlorpromazine (Thorazine®), fluphenazine, and trifluoperazine (Stelazine®); thioxanthines, such as thiothixene (Navane®); butyrophenones, such as haloperidol (Haldol®); and others. These drugs can induce parkinsonism or worsen symptoms of PD.[7] This risk outweighs the potential benefit from this class of drugs, and they should not be used to treat behavioral symptoms in PD. There are six drugs on the US market that are marketed as atypical antipsychotics. These include clozapine (Clozaril®), quetiapine (Seroquel®), risperidone (Risperdal®), olanzapine (Zyprexa®), aripiprazole (Abilify®), and ziprasidone (Geodon®). Atypical antipsychotics are marketed as drugs with good antipsychotic efficacy, but a lower propensity to produce drug-induced parkinsonism and tardive dyskinesia.[8] Clozapine, the prototypic atypical neuroleptic, blocks D_2-like dopamine receptors, but is much more active at the D_4 than at the D_2 and D_3 receptors.[9] The reduced propensity of atypical neuroleptics such as clozapine, to cause parkinsonism may relate to both their reduced affinity for the D_2 receptor and their potent serotonergic blocking activity at the 5-HT_{2A} receptor.[10] Of the other agents, quetiapine most closely resembles clozapine, and may be used in PD. Olanzapine, aripiprazole, and ziprasidone may worsen motor disability and are not currently recommended for use in PD.

Other Neurotransmitters and PD

Acetylcholine

Acetylcholine (ACh) is the neurotransmitter at cholinergic synapses and neuroeffector junctions (eg, muscle, salivary, and sweat glands) in the central and peripheral nervous systems. ACh is synthesized from choline in a reaction controlled by choline acetyltransferase. The actions of ACh are mediated through nicotinic and muscarinic cholinergic receptors.

Muscarinic receptors are found primarily on autonomic effector cells innervated by postganglionic parasympathetic nerves, but are also present in the brain, ganglia, and some cells receiving little or no cholinergic innervation. Pharmacologic study has defined four types of muscarinic receptors: M_1, M_2, M_3, and M_4. A fifth type, defined by using molecular genetics, has not been defined pharmacologically. All muscarinic ACh receptor subtypes interact with a group of guanine nucleotide-binding regulatory proteins (ie, G proteins) that regulate intracellular effector proteins. Activation of muscarinic cholinergic receptors inhibits D_1-like dopamine receptor activation, suggesting ACh antagonism of dopaminergic action.[11] Muscarinic antagonists are used to reduce tremor and rigidity in parkinsonism.

Nicotinic cholinergic receptors mediate neurotransmission at the neuromuscular junction, at autonomic ganglia, and at some CNS sites. Nicotine binding is reduced in the basal ganglia of patients with PD.[12] Nicotinic agonists have been tried in PD, but have been poorly tolerated.

Centrally acting cholinergic agonists include the cholinesterase inhibitors, donepezil (Aricept®), rivastigmine (Exelon®), and galantamine (Razadyne®, Razadyne® ER). Centrally acting cholinergic antagonists include trihexyphenidyl and benztropine (Cogentin®).

Serotonin

Serotonin has been recognized for almost 50 years as an effector on various types of smooth muscle, as an agent that enhances platelet aggregation, and as a CNS neurotransmitter. Serotonin is synthesized from tryptophan in two steps. Tryptophan hydroxylase is the rate-limiting enzyme in serotonin synthesis. The second enzyme, L-aromatic acid hydroxylase, is also important in catecholamine synthesis. Molecular cloning has identified a significant number of serotonin receptor types (at least 15) in four structural and functional families. $5\text{-}HT_1$, $5\text{-}HT_2$, and $5\text{-}HT_4$ receptors are coupled via G proteins to a variety of enzymatic and electric effector systems. The $5\text{-}HT_3$ receptor is a ligand-gated ion channel.

Cerebrospinal fluid (CSF) studies in PD patients suggest reduced amounts of serotonin breakdown products in these patients. Administration of selective serotonin receptor antagonists in animal models of PD potentiates the efficacy of dopaminergic drugs, suggesting that serotonin antagonists might be useful in the therapy of PD.[13] While some studies in levodopa-treated PD patients suggested that depression might correlate with reduced serotonin neurotransmission, a recent study in untreated patients suggested no difference in serotonin metabolites between depressed and nondepressed patients.[14] Serotonergic drugs, such as selective serotonin reuptake inhibitors (SSRIs), have proven useful in the treatment of depression. Concerns that serotonergic drugs might worsen parkinsonism have not been realized.[15]

Glutamate

L-glutamic acid, or glutamate, is the most prevalent excitatory neurotransmitter in the vertebrate nervous system. Glutamate receptors are classified functionally as ligand-gated ion channels or as metabotropic (ie, G-protein coupled) receptors. The ligand-gated ion channels are classified according to the identity of agonists that selectively activate each receptor subtype. These receptors include α-amino-3-hydroxy-5-methyl-4-isoxazole propionic acid (AMPA), kainate, and N-methyl-D-aspartate (NMDA) receptors. AMPA and kainate receptors mediate fast depolarization at most central glutamatergic synapses. NMDA receptors are involved in long-term potentiation and long-term depression, forms of synaptic plasticity. One interesting feature of NMDA receptors is their blockade by Mg^{2+}. Researchers have theorized that cellular energy failure with an inability to maintain the normal resting membrane potential allows the Mg^{2+} to leave its ion channel, rendering the cell vulnerable to glutamate action at the NMDA receptor. Influx of Ca^{2+} into the cell initiates a cascade of events that proves fatal to the cell. This mechanism, dubbed indirect excitotoxicity, has recently been implicated in a number of degenerative nervous system diseases, including PD.[16] Recent or ongoing studies are addressing the question of whether glutamate antagonism might reduce the progression rate of neurodegenerative disease. Riluzole (Rilutek®), lamotrigine (Lamictal®), amantadine (Symmetrel®), and rimantadine (Flumadine®) are marketed agents that have antiglutamatergic activity.

GABA

GABA is the most prevalent inhibitory neurotransmitter in the basal ganglia, where it is important in pathways between the caudate/putamen and globus pallidus, and the globus pallidus pars interna (GPpi) and thalamus. Two types of GABA receptors have been identified. The $GABA_A$ receptor is a ligand-gated Cl^- ion channel. Binding of $GABA$ to this receptor increases chloride influx. This receptor is the site of action of drugs, such as benzodiazepines and barbiturates, as well as the anticonvulsants, topiramate (Topamax®), gabapentin (Neurontin®), and other anticonvulsants. The $GABA_B$ receptor is a member of the G protein-coupled receptor family coupled to biochemical pathways and to the regulation of ion channels. Pharmacologically, baclofen (Kemstro™, Lioresal®) is a $GABA_B$ analogue, and has been useful in the treatment of PD patients with dystonic dyskinesia.

Basal Ganglia Pharmacology and the Future of PD Research

PD can no longer be viewed as a disease of a single chemical neurotransmitter. Evidence is accumulating that the emergence of treatment-related side effects, as well as treatment-resistant symptoms, may relate to interactions among various neurotransmitters. We are just beginning to conduct clinical trials with agents that influence non-dopaminergic neurotransmitter systems, and we are likely to see the benefits of these studies in the near future.

References

1.   Thudichum JL: *A Treatise on the Chemical Constitution of the Brain.* London, England, Balliere, Tindall and Cox, 1884.

2.   Trétiakoff C: *Contribution a l'Etude de l'Anatomie du Locus Niger.* French. These de Paris, Paris, France. 1919.

3.   Kebabian JW: Brain dopamine receptors: 20 years of progress. *Neurochem Res* 1993;18:101-104.

4.   Vingerhoets FJ, Snow BJ, Lee CS, et al: Longitudinal fluorodopa positron emission tomographic studies of the evolution of idiopathic parkinsonism. *Ann Neurol* 1994;36:759-764.

5.   Naidu Y, Chaudhuri KR: Transdermal rotigotine: a new non-ergot dopamine agonist for the treatment of Parkinson's disease. *Expert Opin Drug Deliv* 2007;4:111-118.

6.   Jenner P: The rationale for the use of dopamine agonists in Parkinson's disease. *Neurology* 1995;45(suppl 3):S6-S12.

7.   Grohmann R, Koch R, Schmidt LG: Extrapyramidal symptoms in neuroleptic recipients. *Agents Actions Suppl* 1990;29:71-82.

8.   Factor SA, Brown D, Molho ES, et al: Clozapine: a 2-year open trial in Parkinson's disease patients with psychosis. *Neurology* 1994;44(3 pt 1):544-546.

9.   Seeman P, Van Tol HH: Dopamine receptor pharmacology. *Curr Opin Neurol Neurosurg* 1993;6:602-608.

10.   Meltzer HY: Role of serotonin in the action of atypical antipsychotic drugs. *Clin Neurosci* 1995;3:64-75.

11.   Olianas MC, Onali P: Antagonism of striatal muscarinic receptors inhibiting dopamine D1 receptor-stimulated adenylyl cyclase activity by cholinoceptor antagonist used to treat Parkinson's disease. *Br J Pharmacol* 1996;118:827-828.

12.   Court JA, Piggott MA, Lloyd S: Nicotine binding in human striatum: elevation in schizophrenia and reductions in dementia with Lewy bodies, Parkinson's disease and Alzheimer's disease and in relation to neuroleptic medication. *Neuroscience* 2000;98:79-87.

13.   Fox SH, Moser B, Brotchie JM: Behavioral effects of 5-HT2C receptor antagonism in the substantia nigra zona reticulata of the 6-hydroxydopamine-lesioned rat model of Parkinson's disease. *Exp Neurol* 1998;151:35-49.

14.   Kuhn W, Muller T, Gerlach M, et al: Depression in Parkinson's disease: biogenic amines in CSF of 'de novo' patients. *J Neural Transm* 1996;103:1441-1445.

15.   Zesiewicz TA, Gold M, Chari G et al: Current issues in depression in Parkinson's disease. *Am J Geriatr Psychiatry* 1999;7:110-118.

16.   Beal MF: Mitochondrial dysfunction in neurodegenerative diseases. *Biochim Biophys Acta* 1998;1366:211-223.

Chapter 5

Medical Management of Motor Dysfunction in Early Disease

The goals of medical treatment in early Parkinson's disease (PD) are twofold: to favorably influence disease progression (ie, disease modification) and to maintain functional independence (ie, palliative therapy). Considerable controversy exists about the best way to achieve these goals.

Despite increasing support in laboratory science for putative disease-modifying agents in PD, there is no accepted therapy that alters the disease course. Investigation continues into agents that might influence neurodegeneration by a number of mechanisms, including reducing oxidative processes, blocking excitatory neurotransmission, and improving mitochondrial function.[1,2]

The number of therapeutic agents for the symptomatic treatment of PD continues to grow, but no clear consensus has developed about the optimal agent for early treatment of the disease. At the heart of this controversy is uncertainty about whether levodopa, which is universally acknowledged to dramatically improve the symptoms of the illness, adversely influences the long-term course of PD.

Disease Modification and PD

Efforts to favorably influence the course of PD have been hampered by our incomplete understanding of its etiology and of the mechanisms responsible for progressive cell death in the disease. A number of potentially important factors in neurodegeneration have been identified, including oxidative stress, mitochondrial bioenergetic defects, excitatory neurotransmission, calcium cytotoxicity, and trophin deficiency.[3] The recent discovery of genetic mutations underlying parkinsonism in a small number of families may help to elucidate the basic cellular mechanisms of cell death in PD. Studies in these families suggest that disorders of intracellular protein conformation, handling, or degradation, oxidative stress, and mitochondrial dysfunction are important in PD, but do not yet suggest a therapeutic strategy in familial or sporadic parkinsonism.[4,5]

Animal models have been helpful in studying putative neuroprotective agents, but it is important to remember that PD does not occur in animals. Thus, animal models may not accurately predict clinical benefit. Furthermore, the absence of a widely available biomarker of the disease in humans leads to reliance on clinical measures of disease severity (ie, standardized rating scales). These measures are sensitive to acute and chronic symptomatic medication effects,[6] as well as to the placebo effect.[7] In the most commonly applied strategies to detect a disease-modifying effect, mildly affected PD research subjects who are not yet sufficiently disabled to require potent symptomatic therapies, such as levodopa or dopamine agonists, are randomly assigned a putative neuroprotective agent or a placebo. Subjects are followed for a change in rating scale, such as the Unified Parkinson's Disease Rating Scale (UPDRS) or the time to achieve an end point, such as a need for dopaminergic therapy.[8] The need to distinguish between a palliative effect on the symptoms of PD from a true disease-modifying effect has spurred the development of novel study designs, such as the delayed-start design. In such a study, subjects are randomly assigned to the treatment or placebo for the initial part of the study. After a number of months (usually 6 to 9 months) of blinded treatment, all subjects are placed on the active therapy. This study design aims to account for any symptomatic effect of the study medication. If the experimental intervention exerts only a symptomatic effect, the subjects who start the intervention late should catch up with those who started early. If the intervention has a disease-modifying effect, the group of subjects who took the active agent for the entire duration of the study should be better than those who started it later. Because of the variability of clinical measures of PD, studies of disease modification require several hundred research subjects followed for up to 2 years to demonstrate clinical benefit, and are necessarily expensive.

The largest clinical trial of a neuroprotective agent was the Deprenyl and Tocopherol Antioxidative Therapy of Parkinsonism (DATATOP) study of the selective mono-amine oxidase B (MAO-B) inhibitor selegiline (or deprenyl) and tocopherol. In this study, 801 subjects with early PD who did not require symptomatic therapy were randomly assigned to either: (1) active selegiline (Eldepryl®, Zelapar®) (10 mg/day); (2) active tocopherol (2,000 international units/day); (3) active selegiline and tocopherol; or (4) placebo treatments. Although selegiline delayed the need for levodopa therapy in this study, longer follow-up suggested the effect was not sustained and symptomatic effects of the study intervention confounded our understanding of this effect.[9] In addition, among those patients who reached the end point and were treated with levodopa, disability and complications of levodopa therapy after several years were comparable.[10]

Rasagiline (Azilect®) is a more selective MAO-B inhibitor that is more potent than selegiline. The Trial of Etanercept and Methotrexate with Radiographic Patient Outcomes (TEMPO) study used the delayed-start design to investigate the potential disease-modifying effects of rasagiline. Although research subjects treated with rasagiline for 12 months showed less accrual of disability than those treated only for 6 months, suggesting possible disease modification, a long-term symptomatic effect could not entirely be excluded. A second delayed-start study has been initiated in hopes of duplicating the results of the TEMPO study. Coenzyme Q_{10} is an antioxidant with salutary effects on mitochondrial function. In a small study, subjects with early, untreated PD who were assigned to 1,200 mg daily showed a slower decline in UPDRS score than those assigned to placebo or lower-dose coenzyme Q_{10}.[11] A clinical trial of high-dose coenzyme Q_{10} (2,400 mg/day) is now under way.

Using a novel 'futility' design, the National Institute of Neurological Disorders and Stroke/NIH Exploratory Trials in PD (NINDS/NET-PD) studies suggested that additional study of creatine is warranted.[12]

Despite this increasing evidence base, no disease-modifying therapies for PD can yet be recommended.[13]

Initiation of Symptomatic Therapy

When to begin therapy

The decision to begin symptomatic therapy is based on the joint determination by patient and physician that such treatment is warranted. Both must take into account the disparity between the patient's preserved mobility and the degree of mobility required to maintain a good quality of life. There appears to be little to gain by initiating treatment in a patient who does not consider himself disabled. By the same token, there is little long-term benefit to delaying symptomatic therapy in a patient who is experiencing significant disability.[14] Table 5-1 lists advice on initiating therapy.

Initial therapy

Patients with mild or nondisabling symptoms of PD may benefit from treatment with amantadine or with monoamine oxidase (MAO) inhibitors. Amantadine (Symmetrel®) is an antiviral agent serendipitously noted to have modest anti-parkinsonian effects. Most patients derive adequate benefit from 100 mg twice daily. Younger patients often tolerate 100 mg three times daily. However, amantadine is renally cleared and cautious use in the elderly and in those with known renal insufficiency is warranted. Amantadine may cause livedo

Table 5-1: General Advice About Initiating Therapy

- Discuss therapeutic goals with patients.
- Start dosage low and titrate slowly.
- Teach vocabulary to patients and their families.
- Prescribe an adequate trial of pharmacotherapy.
- When in doubt, schedule a patient visit.

reticularis (ie, a reticular mottling of the skin and limbs), anorexia, nausea, constipation, peripheral edema, confusion, hallucinations, and fatigue. Abrupt withdrawal of amantadine may cause dramatic worsening of parkinsonism.

There are two available selective MAO-B inhibitors, selegiline and rasagiline. Selegiline is available as an oral tablet or capsule (Eldepryl®) and as an orally disintegrating tablet (ODT) (Zelapar®). Selegiline is a suicide inhibitor of MAO-B with extensive first-pass hepatic metabolism and amphetamine metabolites. Selegiline modestly reduces the symptoms of PD in early patients, although it is not US Food and Drug Administration (FDA) approved as monotherapy. Selegiline is given in a dose of 5 mg twice daily. Adverse effects include nausea, dizziness, headache, and insomnia. Selegiline ODT avoids first-pass metabolism and results in much lower levels of amphetamine metabolites. The effects on early PD are similar to the oral preparation. The recommended dose is 1.25 to 2.5 mg dissolved on the tongue once daily. Selegiline ODT is not FDA approved for use as monotherapy in early PD. Rasagiline is a more selective, irreversible MAO-B inhibitor without amphetamine metabolites. Rasagiline is FDA approved as monotherapy for early PD and modestly reduces the severity of PD symptoms. The recommended dose is 1 mg daily. It is well tolerated as monotherapy. MAO inhibitors as a class are contraindicated in patients who are being treated with selective serotonin reuptake inhibitors (SSRIs) and with selective serotonin/norepinephrine reuptake inhibitors (SNRIs) and in those treated with meperidine and other narcotics. ODT selegiline is contraindicated in patients treated with dextromethorphan. Selegiline labeling recommends caution when using the drug with serotonergic as well as with tricyclic antidepressants (TCAs). Rasagiline labeling lists contraindications with cyclobenzaprine, mirtazapine, St. John's wort, dextromethorphan, meperidine and other narcotics, sympathomimetic amines and cautions against use with antidepressants and with foods containing high levels of tyramine.

Anticholinergic medications, such as trihexyphenidyl and benztropine (Cogentin®), are modestly effective for tremor and rigidity in early PD, but are not particularly effective for bradykinesia. In addition, they are difficult to tolerate in therapeutic doses, causing confusion, blurred vision, dry mouth, constipation, and urinary retention. Elderly patients are particularly sensitive to these side effects. Anticholinergic medications may be useful in young, cognitively intact early PD patients with disabling tremor.

If a more potent agent is required from the outset, or if symptoms increase despite the use of minor antiparkinsonian drugs, the physician must choose between carbidopa/levodopa (Sinemet®, Sinemet® CR) and the dopamine agonists bromocriptine (Parlodel®, Parlodel® SnapTabs®), pergolide (Permax®), pramipexole (Mirapex®), and ropinirole (Requip®). Pergolide products have been withdrawn from the US market due to concerns about cardiac valvulopathy, but they remain available outside the United States. The ideal initial drug for PD should have the following characteristics: (1) it should reproduce the natural pattern of dopamine stimulation of postsynaptic receptors; (2) it should be highly effective for long-term use; (3) it should be well tolerated; (4) it should not contribute to the degenerative process; and (5) it should be reasonably priced. Unfortunately, no single agent meets all of these exacting criteria.

Carbidopa/levodopa remains the most commonly pre-scribed, potent therapeutic agent for PD. The drug combines levodopa, the precursor of dopamine, with carbidopa, an aromatic acid decarboxylase inhibitor that decreases the peripheral conversion of levodopa to dopamine, increasing brain levodopa levels and decreasing dopaminergic peripheral side effects. This results in dopamine receptor stimulation. Carbidopa/levodopa is highly effective. Indeed, it so dramatically improves all of the cardinal signs of the illness that levodopa responsiveness has become one of the diagnostic criteria for the disease. It is also well tolerated and reasonably priced.

However, not long after levodopa became available, its shortcomings became apparent. After several years of therapy, patients developed progressive shortening of the duration of benefit after a single dose ('wearing-off' phenomenon). Some patients developed unpredictable medication responses, such as sudden and extreme fluctuations in motor function, including severe akinesia, despite adequate plasma levodopa levels ('on-off' syndrome). In addition, different types of involuntary movements (ie, dyskinesias) developed, and patients began to complain of sleep disorders, hallucinations, and psychosis.

Evidence began to accumulate that oxidative mechanisms in the brain might contribute to the degenerative process, and some postulated that the ability of levodopa to generate reactive oxygen species might make it toxic to brain cells. Some physicians began to recommend delaying the use of levodopa until patients were significantly disabled. Retrospective studies of dopamine agonists suggested they may protect against the development of motor fluctuations and these were suggested as an alternative to levodopa for initial therapy.

Which drug is best suited for initiation of potent symp-tomatic therapy in PD remains the most critical controversy in the field. The main issues are (1) whether carbidopa/levodopa contributes to the degenerative process in PD, and (2) whether levodopa contributes to the development of motor fluctuations and dyskinesia in treated patients.

Does levodopa contribute to the degenerative process in PD?

Despite laboratory evidence that the oxidative metabolism of levodopa may harm neurons,[15,16] there is no clinical evidence that levodopa unfavorably influences the disease course in PD. Levodopa therapy prolongs life expectancy in PD. The Parkinson Study Group randomly assigned 361 subjects with early, untreated PD to placebo or one of three doses of carbidopa/levodopa (Early vs Late Levodopa in Parkinson's Disease [ELLDOPA] study). Subjects were evaluated for more than 40 weeks, then following a 2-week withdrawal period. Subjects randomly assigned to placebo declined more from baseline to the end of washout than did subjects in the levodopa groups, suggesting either a disease-modifying effect or a prolonged symptomatic effect, but not that levodopa is toxic in early PD.[17]

Does levodopa contribute to the development of motor fluctuations and dyskinesia in levodopa-treated patients?

In the normal physiologic state, dopamine receptors are tonically stimulated. Accumulating evidence suggests that the pulsatile stimulation of dopamine receptors that is characteristic of levodopa with its short half-life, contributes both to the progressive development of motor response fluctuations and to the development of peak-dose dyskinesia.[18] The longer duration of receptor stimulation produced by drugs with longer half-lives, such as dopamine agonists, may protect against the development of motor response fluctuations. Historically, dopamine agonist monotherapy has almost never been associated with the development of dyskinesias or motor response fluctuations.[19] Studies have shown that the development of motor response fluctuations is reduced by initial treatment with a dopamine agonist.[19-22] Those fluctuations include shortening of duration of response to individual doses of the drug between doses ('wearing-off' phenomenon), sudden and unpredictable loss of motor efficacy ('on-off' syndrome), and dyskinesias. Two recently published, randomized, double-blind studies comparing carbidopa/levodopa with ropinirole[20] or pramipexole[21] are worth specific mention. In both studies, early PD patients were randomly assigned to treatment with a dopamine agonist or with carbidopa/levodopa. After the initial dose titration phase, supplementation with open-label carbidopa/levodopa was allowed. Initiating antiparkinsonian therapy with a dopamine agonist reduced the development of dyskinesia by 67% at 2 years and 60% at 4 years in the pramipexole study and by 50% in the 5-year ropinirole study. The development of shortened response duration after a single dose and unpredictable loss of response occurred more often with levodopa than with pramipexole at 2 years, although there was no difference in the 5-year ropinirole study. The drawbacks to initiation of symptomatic therapy with dopamine agonists were well illustrated in the studies. Both showed that the antiparkinsonian effect was significantly less for the agonist than for carbidopa/levodopa. Hallucinations were about three times as likely in the agonist treatment groups (9% vs 3% at 2 years with pramipexole, and 17% vs 6% at 5 years with ropinirole). Somnolence was also more common in the agonist treatment arms of both studies. Other rare, but potentially disabling complications of dopamine agonist therapy include peripheral edema, fibrotic valvulopathy (with ergot-derived agents—pergolide and bromocriptine) and compulsive behaviors, such as gambling, shopping, eating, hypersexuality, and others.[23] In clinical practice, dopamine agonist monotherapy is significantly more expensive than carbidopa/levodopa monotherapy.

These studies suggest that initiation of therapy for PD with a dopamine agonist might confer protection against the development of dyskinesia and perhaps motor fluctuations, at least in the short term, but that dopamine agonists are less efficacious and more difficult to tolerate than levodopa.

It is important to remember that the symptomatic treatment of PD continues for decades. It remains to be seen whether the initial choice of antiparkinsonian agent determines the state of the patient at 10 or 15 years of therapy, when therapy for most patients becomes difficult and quality of life is substantially reduced. It is also worth remembering that participants in clinical trials tend to be younger and healthier than the general clinic population. Therapy should be directed by the clinical state of the individual patient, depending on the need for greater efficacy and tolerability (better with levodopa) or the desire to delay the onset of motor complications (better with dopamine agonists). Because younger patients are more prone to develop motor fluctuations and more likely to tolerate agonists, many clinicians begin treatment with agonists in all patients younger than age 60 and many between the ages of 60 and 70. The presence of significant cognitive impairment is usually considered a contraindication to dopamine agonist monotherapy.

How to Initiate Therapy With Dopaminergic Drugs
Carbidopa/levodopa

Carbidopa/levodopa is available in a standard-release form (Sinemet®), a controlled-release form (Sinemet® CR), and a fixed-dose combination with entacapone (Stalevo®). Standard-release carbidopa/levodopa contains the peripheral aromatic acid decarboxylase inhibitor carbidopa and levodopa in a ratio of 1:10 (carbidopa/levodopa 10/100 or 25/250 mg) or 1:4 (carbidopa/levodopa 25/100 mg). It is generally administered 3 to 4 times daily in early PD. Controlled-release carbidopa/levodopa contains carbidopa and levodopa in the 1:4 ratio (25/100 or 50/200), but is formulated as a slowly eroding matrix. This contributes to a delayed onset of therapeutic benefit after a single dose, but prolongs the duration of benefit from that dose. Controlled-release carbidopa/levodopa can be administered twice daily in early PD. Because a drug with a longer duration of action should lessen the development of motor fluctuations and dyskinesia, one might assume that the controlled-release preparation is superior to the standard preparation of carbidopa/levodopa. However, a study comparing the standard-release form (Sinemet®) to the controlled-release form (Sinemet® CR) failed to demonstrate a difference in the development of motor response fluctuations between the treatment groups. Both drugs were effective for the 5-year study period. The study did show that the group treated with controlled-release carbidopa/levodopa had better function on scales measuring activities of daily living, but not on measures of motor function.[24] Carbidopa/levodopa/entacapone (Stalevo®) is available in three dose strengths: 12.5/50/200, 25/100/200, and 37.5/150/200 mg. It is not currently indicated for the treatment of early PD.

Most patients require 75 to 100 mg of carbidopa daily to block peripheral conversion of levodopa to dopamine. Because peripheral metabolism of levodopa to dopamine both reduces the amount of levodopa available to the brain and contributes to adverse effects such as nausea, vomiting, and orthostatic hypotension, it is often best to maximize the carbidopa dose in early disease by using a 1:4 carbidopa to levodopa ratio. Pure carbidopa 25 mg can be added to increase the total carbidopa dose to block peripheral degradation of levodopa.

Carbidopa/levodopa is usually started at a dose of 150 to 200 mg levodopa daily. Standard carbidopa/levodopa can be started at a dose of 25/100 mg, one-half tablet three times daily, and controlled-release carbidopa/levodopa can be started at a dose of 25/100 mg twice daily. The dose is then titrated gradually as tolerated by the patient. A titration rate of 50 to 100 mg levodopa/week is usually adequate and well tolerated. Many patients need between 300 and 600 mg levodopa/day to treat disability in early disease. The clinician should probably see the patient in person before recommending an increase in levodopa dose above 600 mg/day. There is no absolute maximum dose of carbidopa/levodopa, but it is unusual for a patient with early PD to require doses in excess of 600 mg levodopa daily.

Dopamine agonists: bromocriptine, pergolide, pramipexole, roprinirole, and rotigotine

Five dopamine agonists are approved for the treatment of PD: bromocriptine (Parlodel®, Parlodel® SnapTabs®), pergolide (Permax®), pramipexole (Mirapex®), ropinirole (Requip®), and the rotigotine transdermal patch (Neupro®). Pergolide was withdrawn voluntarily from the US market due to concerns about fibrotic valvulopathy in treated patients, but pergolide is still available outside the United States. Cabergoline has been studied in PD, but is marketed for the treatment of prolactinoma, and its use in PD is prohibitively expensive[25] (Table 5-2). A recent multicenter randomized, double-blind, placebo-controlled study of the rotigotine transdermal patch showed significant improvements in motor scores and activities of daily living.

Although only pramipexole, ropinirole, and rotigotine are labeled for use as monotherapy in early PD, all agonists have been studied and shown efficacious in this population. Bromocriptine and pergolide are ergot-derived agents, which may contribute to a greater incidence of vascular and other side effects. Pulmonary and retroperitoneal fibrosis and fibrotic valvulopathy have also been reported with ergot-derived dopamine agonists and prompted the voluntary withdrawl of pergolide from the US market.[26,27] Although pulmonary and retroperitoneal fibrosis are rare, recent studies suggest a sevenfold increase in the risk of fibrotic valvulopathy in patients treated with ergot-derived dopamine agonists.[28] An anecdotal report suggested an association between pramipexole and 'sleep attacks,' resulting in several automobile accidents.[29] However, sedation is known to occur in PD itself and to complicate therapy with all antiparkinsonian agents. The relative risk of sedation among antiparkinsonian agents is unknown.

Table 5-2: Initial Dose and Subsequent Titration of Dopamine Agonists

Drug	Initial Dose/ Titration	Therapeutic Range
Bromocriptine (Parlodel®, Parlodel® SnapTabs®)	1.25 mg b.i.d., increase by 2.5 mg every 14-18 days	15 to 40 mg/d
Pergolide (Permax®)*	0.05 mg daily, increase by 0.1 to 0.15 mg/d q3d × 12 days then may increase by 0.25 mg q3d	2 to 5 mg/d
Pramipexole (Mirapex®)	0.125 mg t.i.d., increase by 0.125 mg/dose in week 2 and 0.25 mg/ dose in weeks 3-7	1.5 to 4.5 mg/d
Ropinirole (Requip®)	0.25 mg t.i.d., increase by 0.25 mg/dose weekly × 4 weeks	4.5 to 24 mg/d
Rotigotine transdermal patch (Neupro®)	2 mg/24 hr, increase by 2 mg weekly	4-6 mg/24 hr
Cabergoline**	0.25 mg, increase by 0.25 mg weekly	0.25 to 4 mg/d

*Pergolide (Permax®) and its generic products were voluntarily withdrawn from the US market.

**Not FDA approved for the treatment of Parkinson's disease.

Each dopamine agonist has its own unique profile of activity at different subtypes of the dopamine receptors. In this sense, none stimulates dopamine receptors in the same physiologic way as natural dopamine. However, all have a longer half-life than levodopa, so they more closely model the tonic receptor stimulation profile that appears to be important in the avoidance of motor fluctuations and dyskinesia. Although all available dopamine agonists have shown efficacy during long-term use, the magnitude of response to dopamine agonists is less than that for carbidopa/levodopa. Dopamine agonists are less well tolerated than carbidopa/levodopa, and therapy with dopamine agonists is more expensive than therapy with carbidopa/levodopa.

Common side effects of direct-acting dopamine agonists include nausea, vomiting, constipation, headache, dizziness or symptomatic orthostatic hypotension, fatigue, somnolence, hallucinations, and edema. Rotigotine use may also be associated with skin reactions at the application site. Many patients who begin therapy with direct-acting dopamine agonists complain that their parkinsonian symptoms are worse during the early phase of drug titration. This appears to result from preferential stimulation of dopamine receptors on the presynaptic neuron, decreasing dopamine release from the neurons. Patients should be counseled that their symptoms may worsen slightly before improving, and that they should avoid discontinuing the drug until therapeutic levels are reached. There have been few direct comparisons of the efficacy and toxicity of individual dopamine agonists.

Bromocriptine is an ergot-derived dopamine agonist that is approved by the FDA as an adjunctive agent for the treatment of PD. Its half-life is 12 to 15 hours. Several small studies suggest efficacy as monotherapy in early PD.[30] The initial dose of bromocriptine is 1.25 mg once daily. The dose can be increased by 1.25 mg every 3 to 7 days until a target dose of 15 to 40 mg is achieved. The risk of fibrotic valvulopathy dictates extreme caution in the use of this ergot-based agent.

Pergolide is a semisynthetic ergot-derived dopamine agonist that is approved by the FDA as an adjunctive agent for the treatment of PD. Its half-life is 24 hours. Double-blind, placebo-controlled studies suggest it is also useful as monotherapy in PD.[31] The recommended titration of pergolide begins with 0.05 mg daily for 2 days, followed by incremental increases of 0.1 to 0.15 mg every 3 days as tolerated for 12 days. The dose can be increased by increments of 0.25 mg/day every 3 days thereafter, to a final dose range of 2 to 5 mg/day. The risk of fibrotic valvulopathy dictates extreme caution in the use of this ergot-based agent. Pergolide is no longer available in the United States, but remains available in other countries.

Pramipexole is a nonergot dopamine agonist that is approved by the FDA as monotherapy in early PD and as adjunctive therapy in advanced PD.[32] Its half-life ranges from 8 to 12 hours. The initial dose of pramipexole is 0.125 mg, three times daily. The dose is increased to 0.25 mg three times daily in week one, then to 0.5 mg three times daily in week two. Subsequent increases of 0.25 mg/dose can be made as needed. However, dose-response curves in one study suggested that dose increases above 1.5 mg daily may not improve efficacy.[33] The dose of pramipexole must be adjusted in patients with renal impairment.

Ropinirole is a nonergot dopamine agonist that is aproved by the FDA as monotherapy or as adjunctive therapy of PD.[32] Titration of ropinirole begins with 0.25 mg three times daily. The dose is increased by 0.25 mg/dose to 0.5 mg three times daily in week one, 0.75 mg three times daily in week two, and 1 mg three times daily in week three, followed by 0.5 mg/dose increases to a maximum dose of 24 mg/day.

Rotigotine is a nonergot dopamine agonist that is available as a transdermal patch (Neupro®). The recommended initial dose is 2 mg (10 cm²) increasing weekly as tolerated to 6 mg daily (30 cm²) per 24 hours. The patch is applied to hairless skin, rotating the application site daily.

Cabergoline is a long-acting, ergot-derived dopamine receptor agonist approved by the FDA for the treatment of prolactinoma, but not for PD. It is priced accordingly, and is prohibitively expensive for use in PD. However, placebo-controlled trials confirm that cabergoline is safe and effective as monotherapy in PD. It has the longest half-life of any available dopaminergic agonist (65 hours). Cabergoline can be started at a dose of 0.25 mg daily. The dose can be increased by 0.25 mg daily every week, to a range of 0.25 to 4 mg daily.

Following Patients With Early PD on Dopaminergic Therapy

Most patients with early PD can be seen in the office or outpatient clinic every 4 to 6 months. For average patients, good control is achieved using monotherapy or combined therapy with levodopa or dopamine agonists. These patients have a stable course for several years and do not require complicated drug regimens. It is important from the outset that the goals of therapy be realistic. If the patient or physician aims for complete control of symptoms, adverse effects are likely. The goal of therapy should be functional independence, and the level of function required to achieve this varies significantly from person to person. Drug titration is most successful if drugs are started in a dose as low as possible, titrated very slowly, and given adequate time to produce a therapeutic effect. Generally, a therapeutic trial should last at least 30 days on a stable dose in the drug's selected therapeutic range. The patient should be educated about the disease and the drug's expected beneficial and harmful effects. It is wise to begin to introduce terms such as 'wearing-off' and 'dyskinesia' so that the physician and patient use the same vocabulary to describe emerging symptoms. At follow-up visits, the physician should also ask about concomitant medications, sleep disruption, excessive daytime sleepiness, cognitive dysfunction or confusion, depression, hallucinations, edema, cardiac symptoms, obsessive or repetitive behaviors, and other changes. Supine and standing blood pressures should be checked.

Unfortunately, the stable response to dopaminergic therapy wanes. Most patients take levodopa alone or in combination with a dopamine agonist by the fifth year of therapy, and most will begin to notice minor changes in response to therapy. Typically, these include wearing off of benefit between doses or the occurrence of dyskinesia at the peak of medication effect. While these minor annoyances can be treated by adjusting the incremental levodopa dose and interdose interval, or by adding adjunctive agents, they signal the transition to a more complicated therapeutic regimen and diminishing satisfaction with PD symptom control.

References

1.   Olanow CW: Attempts to obtain neuroprotection in Parkinson's disease. *Neurology* 1997;49(suppl 1):S26-S33.

2.   Simon DK, Standaert DG: Neuroprotective therapies. *Med Clin North Am* 1999;83:509-523.

3.   Olanow CW: A scientific rationale for protective therapy in Parkinson's disease. *J Neural Transm Gen Sect* 1993;91:161-180.

4.   Abbas N, Lucking CB, Ricard S, et al: A wide variety of mutations in the parkin gene are responsible for autosomal recessive parkinsonism in Europe. French Parkinson's Disease Genetics Study Group and the European Consortium on Genetic Susceptibility in Parkinson's Disease. *Hum Mol Genet* 1999;8:567-574.

5.   Polymeropoulos MH: Autosomal dominant Parkinson's disease and alpha-synuclein. *Ann Neurol* 1998;44(3 suppl 1):S63-S64.

6.   Ward CD: Does selegiline delay progression of Parkinson's disease? A critical re-evaluation of the DATATOP study. *J Neurol Neurosurg Psychiatry* 1994;57:217-220.

7.   Goetz CG, Leurgans S, Raman R, et al: Objective changes in motor function during placebo treatment in PD. *Neurology* 2000;54: 710-714.

8.   Fahn S, Elton RL, Committee UD: Unified Parkinson's disease rating scale. In: Fahn S, Marsden CD, Goldstein, et al, eds: *Recent Developments in Parkinson's Disease*. New York, NY, Macmillan, 1987, pp 153-163.

9.   Parkinson Study Group: Impact of deprenyl and tocopherol treatment on Parkinson's disease in DATATOP subjects not requiring levodopa. *Ann Neurol* 1996;39:29-36.

10.   Parkinson Study Group: Impact of deprenyl and tocopherol treatment on Parkinson's disease in DATATOP patients requiring levodopa. *Ann Neurol* 1996;39:37-45.

11.   Shults CW, Oakes D, Kieburtz K, et al: Effects of coenzyme Q10 in early Parkinson disease: evidence of slowing of the functional decline. *Arch Neurol* 2002;59:1541-1550.

12.   NET-PD Investigators: A randomized, double-blind, futility clinical trial of creatine and minocycline in early Parkinson disease. *Neurology* 2006;66:664-671.

13.   Suchowersky O, Gronseth G, Perlmutter J, et al: Practice Parameter: neuroprotective strategies and alternative therapies for Parkinson disease (an evidence-based review). Report of the Quality Standards Subcommittee of the American Academy of Neurology. *Neurology* 2006;66:976-982.

14.   Fahn S: Parkinson disease, the effect of levodopa, and the ELLDOPA trial. Earlier vs Later L-DOPA. *Arch Neurol* 1999;56: 529-535.

15.   Hirsch EC: Does oxidative stress participate in nerve cell death in Parkinson's disease? *Eur Neurol* 1993;33(suppl 1):52-59.

16.   Olanow C: A rationale for dopamine agonists as primary therapy for Parkinson's disease. *Can J Neurol Sci* 1992;19(1 suppl): 108-112.

17.   Fahn S, Oakes D, Shoulson I, et al: Levodopa and the progression of Parkinson's disease. *N Engl J Med* 2004;351:2498-2508.

18.   Chase TN: Levodopa therapy: consequences of the nonphysiologic replacement of dopamine. *Neurology* 1998;50(5 suppl 5) S17-S25.

19.   Rinne UK, Bracco F, Chouza C, et al: Early treatment of Parkinson's disease with cabergoline delays the onset of motor complications. Results of a double-blind levodopa controlled trial. The PKDS009 Study Group. *Drugs* 1998;55(suppl 1):23-30.

20.   Rascol O, Brooks DJ, Korczyn AD, et al: A five-year study of the incidence of dyskinesia in patients with early Parkinson's disease who were treated with ropinirole or levodopa. 056 Study Group. *N Engl J Med* 2000;342:1484-1491.

21.   Parkinson Study Group: Pramipexole vs levodopa as initial treatment for Parkinson Disease. A randomized controlled trial. *JAMA* 2000;284:1931-1938.

22.   Holloway RG, Shoulson I, Fahn S, et al: Pramipexole vs levodopa as initial treatment for Parkinson disease: a 4-year randomized controlled trial. *Arch Neurol* 2004;61:1044-1053.

23.   Voon V, Hassan K, Zurowski M, et al: Prospective prevalence of pathologic gambling and medication association in Parkinson disease. *Neurology* 2006;66:1750-1752.

24.   Block G, Liss C, Reines S, et al: Comparison of immediate-release and controlled release carbidopa/levodopa in Parkinson's disease. A multicenter 5-year study. The CR First Study Group. *Eur Neurol* 1997;37:23-27.

25.   Fariello RG: Pharmacodynamic and pharmacokinetic features of cabergoline. Rationale for use in Parkinson's disease. *Drugs* 1998; 55(suppl 1):10-16.

26.   Klaassen RJ, Troost RJ, Verhoeven GT, et al: Suggestive evidence for bromocriptine-induced pleurisy. *Neth J Med* 1996;48:232-236.

27.   Jimenez-Jimenez FJ, Lopez-Alvarez J, Sanchez-Chapado M, et al: Retroperitoneal fibrosis in a patient with Parkinson's disease treated with pergolide. *Clin Neuropharmacol* 1995;18:277-279.

28.   Schade R, Andersohn F, Suissa S, et al: Dopamine agonists and the risk of cardiac-valve regurgitation. *N Engl J Med* 2007;356:29-38.

29.   Frucht S, Rogers JD, Greene PE, et al: Falling asleep at the wheel: motor vehicle mishaps in persons taking pramipexole and ropinirole. *Neurology* 1999;52:1908-1910.

30.   Nakanishi T, Kanazawa I, Iwata M, et al: Nation-wide collaborative study on the long-term effects of bromocriptine in the treatment of parkinsonian patients: analysis on the maintenance and the change of the original mode of treatment. *Eur Neurol* 1992;32(suppl 1):23-29.

31.   Kulisevsky J, Lopez-Villegas D, Garcia-Sanchez C, et al: A six-month study of pergolide and levodopa in de novo Parkinson's disease patients. *Clin Neuropharmacol* 1998;21:358-362.

32.   Pramipexole and ropinirole for Parkinson's disease. *Med Lett Drugs Ther* 1997;39:109-110.

33.   Safety and efficacy of pramipexole in early Parkinson's disease. A randomized dose-ranging study. Parkinson Study Group. *JAMA* 1997;278:125-130.

Chapter 6

Medical Management of Motor Dysfunction in Moderate-to-Advanced Disease

n its early stages, Parkinson's disease (PD) is a forgiving illness. Once the obstacles of identification, accurate diagnosis, and deciding the appropriate time and type of initial therapy have been overcome, therapy proceeds smoothly for several years. Rapid progression and the development of severe side effects are so rare during the first 5 years that they call into question the accuracy of diagnosis. The characteristics of the transition from mild PD to moderate-to-advanced PD are the loss of smooth response to dopaminergic therapy with the development of motor fluctuations; the emergence and progression of levodopa-resistant symptoms; and the occurrence in many patients of adverse psychiatric effects of therapy (see Chapter 8) and cognitive decline. Most patients begin to experience inconsistencies in their response to medications after about 5 years of levodopa therapy, but they may occur earlier, particularly in patients whose disease begins before 40 years of age, and later in patients who have been treated initially with dopamine agonist monotherapy (see Chapter 5).

Typically, patients first notice motor fluctuations. These represent a deterioration in the seamless response to therapy to which they have become accustomed and are usually associated with dyskinesias (ie, abnormal involuntary movements).[1] Later, levodopa-resistant symptoms emerge, such as freezing during periods of good motor function, and levodopa-resistant speech and swallowing deterioration. Finally, a significant minority of patients develop drug-induced confusion, hallucinations, and even psychosis, which will be addressed in Chapter 8.

Motor Fluctuations

Motor fluctuations related to levodopa dose

Early in the course of levodopa therapy, patients have a 'long-duration response.' The drug can be taken three times daily with a smooth antiparkinsonian response; when the drug is discontinued, it takes days or weeks for the patient to achieve maximal immobility.[2] Levodopa also has a short-duration response lasting minutes to hours, which is more consistent with its short plasma half-life and is not apparent in early treatment.[2] However, with disease evolution, the short-duration response becomes more prominent. In addition, the response profile takes on an all-or-none quality with a threshold for efficacy. If the threshold is not reached, there is no benefit from the dose (ie, dose failure). When the threshold is met, symptoms improve. Exceeding the threshold does not increase the magnitude of benefit, but it does prolong the duration of benefit.[3] Doses over the threshold may be associated with dyskinesia, involuntary choreic movements, or involuntary dystonic movements.

Further increasing the incremental dose over the threshold for the production of dyskinesia prolongs the duration of dyskinesia, but does not increase its magnitude. The separation between the threshold for antiparkinsonian response and that for dyskinesia is relatively wide in early PD, so that it takes doses much larger than those associated with antiparkinsonian benefit to produce dyskinesia. However, the pulsatile nature of dopamine receptor stimulation produces actual changes in the dopamine receptors that lower the threshold for dyskinesia production, so that in advanced PD, the dyskinesia threshold may be just barely above, or even below, that required for antiparkinsonian benefit.[4]

Most motor fluctuations in PD are related to difficulty in delivering dopamine to its striatal receptors. Dopamine delivery to the receptor is a multistep process: the pill must be taken, the levodopa must be absorbed, levodopa must be protected from degradation before it crosses the blood-brain barrier, it must be converted into dopamine in the presynaptic neuron, released at the presynaptic terminal, and bind to the dopamine receptor (Figure 6-1). Failure in any of these steps produces dose-related motor fluctuations, which include fluctuations related to delayed gastric emptying or competition with dietary amino acids, premature wearing-off, and dose failure. Attention to motor fluctuations in PD is important because fluctuations significantly degrade patient quality of life. [5]

Wearing-off, or end-of-dose deterioration, refers to a loss of levodopa effect before the next dose is given. Significant wearing-off develops in 20% to 50% of patients after 5 years of levodopa therapy.[6] Most patients first experience this phenomenon when they need to take an afternoon dose before its scheduled time or when stiffness and slowness reappear in the morning before the first dose of levodopa.[7] Later, parkinsonian bradykinesia or tremor recurs before each dose. This wearing-off between doses is first noticed at about 4 hours after the dose, but the duration of response shortens to 3, 2, or even 1 hour as the disease progresses. As wearing-off worsens, the rapidity of deterioration at the end of the dose interval increases, and patients often complain that they go from mobile to immobile in only seconds, as if a light switch were turned off.

Changes in absorption of levodopa contribute to these fluctuations. Levodopa is absorbed in the small bowel by the facilitated transport mechanism. Delayed emptying of the stomach into the small bowel caused by degeneration of neurons in the intestinal wall may produce a lower-than-

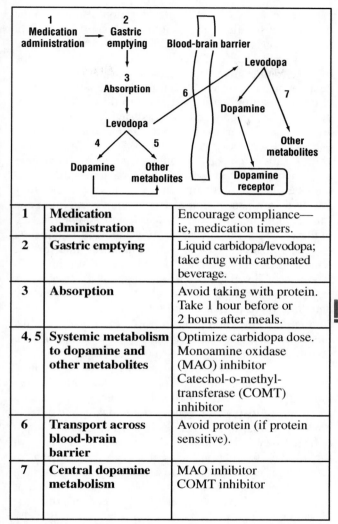

1	**Medication administration**	Encourage compliance—ie, medication timers.
2	**Gastric emptying**	Liquid carbidopa/levodopa; take drug with carbonated beverage.
3	**Absorption**	Avoid taking with protein. Take 1 hour before or 2 hours after meals.
4, 5	**Systemic metabolism to dopamine and other metabolites**	Optimize carbidopa dose. Monoamine oxidase (MAO) inhibitor Catechol-o-methyl-transferase (COMT) inhibitor
6	**Transport across blood-brain barrier**	Avoid protein (if protein sensitive).
7	**Central dopamine metabolism**	MAO inhibitor COMT inhibitor

Figure 6-1: Steps in dopamine delivery to the dopamine receptor, and potential interventions to maximize delivery.

6

expected plasma level, a shorter-duration response to the dose, or a dose failure. The facilitated transport mechanism for levodopa is also responsible for the absorption of large neutral amino acids. If a dose is taken too close in time to protein ingestion, the subsequent plasma peak may be delayed or reduced, which can produce delayed onset of effect, premature wearing-off, or frank dose failure. Levodopa can be metabolized in the systemic circulation by aromatic acid decarboxylase, monoamine oxidase (MAO), or catechol-o-methyltransferase (COMT). The large neutral amino acid/levodopa-facilitated transport mechanism is also important in transport of levodopa across the blood-brain barrier, and circulating large neutral amino acids may interfere with penetration of levodopa into the brain and cause additional havoc with drug response.[8] When several of these factors—including a barely adequate incremental levodopa dose, delayed stomach emptying, interference with absorption by a large protein load, and systemic metabolism of levodopa—exist simultaneously, a complex response to levodopa can occur, with unpredictable onset and duration of response, and dose failures.

Studies on the pathogenesis of wearing-off suggest that this phenomenon is not related simply to a change in drug pharmacokinetics, but rather, to central mechanisms. The presence of wearing-off best correlates with the duration of PD, suggesting that loss of presynaptic dopamine nerve terminals is important. In clinical studies, continuous intravenous infusions of levodopa dramatically and quickly ameliorate wearing-off, suggesting that a failure of dopamine delivery to the brain is also important in the genesis of the response fluctuation.[9] Thus, it appears that wearing-off reflects the degeneration of dopamine terminals because of disease progression with reduced ability to buffer variations in plasma levodopa levels, and receptor changes that lead to increased dependence on stable plasma levels. Because levodopa has a short plasma half-life (ie, about 2 hours), it is difficult to produce stable levels.[9]

Motor fluctuations unrelated to levodopa dose

About 10% of patients complain of sudden changes in mobility occurring at unexpected times (based on the dose interval or on protein ingestion [ie, 'on-off' syndrome]). In such patients, short-term continuous infusions of levodopa do not reverse the off periods, suggesting that poor drug delivery is not the reason for the change in mobility.[4] Researchers believe that postsynaptic changes in the receptors themselves or downstream mechanisms are responsible for these fluctuations.[10] 'On-off' syndrome is also related to disease duration. Most patients with 'on-off' syndrome also have wearing-off and protein-related 'off' periods, creating a complicated response pattern that can vary considerably from day to day. Only careful study of 'on-off' diaries reveals which off periods can successfully be remedied by better drug delivery (Figure 6-2).

Dyskinesia
Definitions and natural history of dyskinesia

The term dyskinesia encompasses several different types of involuntary movement (Table 6-1). Dyskinesias can be classified by the type of movement and the phase of drug response in which they occur. Movement types include chorea, dystonia, myoclonus, and tic.[11] Movements occur during on time (ie, peak-dose dyskinesia), during the transition between on and off (ie, diphasic dyskinesia), and during off time (ie, 'off'-period dyskinesia).

Chorea, which comes from the Greek word for 'dance,' is the most common involuntary movement associated with the treatment of PD. Choreic movements are random, rapid, purposeless, writhing that typically occur at the peak of levodopa effect, and comprise part of the peak-dose dyskinesia syndrome. Patients are often not aware of early chorea, and chorea is generally not seen in patients on dopamine agonist monotherapy.

Dystonia is a slower, twisting, patterned movement, and is frequently painful. Dystonia may be part of the underlying

'On-Off' Diary

Instructions: For each hour of the day and night, circle the state that best describes your physical function over the *preceding* hour. Record the dose and time of any levodopa taken in that hour as well.

Drug/time	Time	
	Midnight	off
	1:00 AM	off
	2:00 AM	off
	3:00 AM	off
	4:00 AM	off
	5:00 AM	off
	6:00 AM	off
	7:00 AM	off
	8:00 AM	off
	9:00 AM	off
	10:00 AM	off
	11:00 AM	off
	Noon	off
	1:00 PM	off
	2:00 PM	off
	3:00 PM	off
	4:00 PM	off
	5:00 PM	off
	6:00 PM	off
	7:00 PM	off
	8:00 PM	off
	9:00 PM	off
	10:00 PM	off
	11:00 PM	off

Figure 6-2: Sample of an 'on-off' diary for patients.

Off=stiff and slow, feeling no benefit from your medications

On=loose and able to move about, feeling good benefit from your medications

On with dyskinesia=loose and able to move about, feeling good benefit from your medications, but with superimposed twisting or writhing movements (not rhythmic tremor)

on	on with dyskinesia	asleep
on	on with dyskinesia	asleep
on	on with dyskinesia	asleep
on	on with dyskinesia	asleep
on	on with dyskinesia	asleep
on	on with dyskinesia	asleep
on	on with dyskinesia	asleep
on	on with dyskinesia	asleep
on	on with dyskinesia	asleep
on	on with dyskinesia	asleep
on	on with dyskinesia	asleep
on	on with dyskinesia	asleep
on	on with dyskinesia	asleep
on	on with dyskinesia	asleep
on	on with dyskinesia	asleep
on	on with dyskinesia	asleep
on	on with dyskinesia	asleep
on	on with dyskinesia	asleep
on	on with dyskinesia	asleep
on	on with dyskinesia	asleep
on	on with dyskinesia	asleep
on	on with dyskinesia	asleep
on	on with dyskinesia	asleep
on	on with dyskinesia	asleep
on	on with dyskinesia	asleep

6

Table 6-1: Treatment of Motor Fluctuations

Motor Complication	Treatment Alternatives
Wearing-off	Use smaller incremental dose, more frequent administration.
	Change to controlled-release carbidopa/levodopa (Sinemet® CR).
	Add amantadine (Symmetrel®), entacapone (COMTan®), tolcapone (Tasmar®), rasagiline (Azilect®), selegiline (Eldepryl®, Zelapar®).
	Add dopamine agonist.
	Use liquid levodopa.
On-off	Characterize problem with 'on-off' diaries.
	Treat 'wearing-off', protein-related 'off', and dose failure components.
	Add dopamine agonist.
Protein-related 'off'	Reduce daytime protein.
	Balanced 7:1 carbohydrate-to-protein ratio.
Peak-dose dyskinesia	Reduce incremental dose, but watch for increased wearing-off.
	Use liquid levodopa.
'Off'-period dystonia	Use controlled-release levodopa.
	Add dopamine agonist.
Diphasic dyskinesia	Maximize 'on' time.
	Use liquid levodopa.

disease, and patients may complain of clawing or gripping movements of the more involved foot, even in the absence of symptomatic treatment. Dystonia may accompany chorea at the peak of medication effect. Pure dystonia in treated PD tends to present as painful foot and leg cramping in the early morning before the first daily levodopa dose. It may awaken the patient from sleep, but tends to be transient, disappearing about 45 minutes after it begins, or more promptly if the patient takes his or her regular dose of levodopa.

Myoclonus and tics are rapid, usually simple movements that are seen during the 'on' state and make up part of the peak-dose dyskinesia syndrome.

During the transition periods between 'on' and 'off' states, some patients develop stereotypical kicking movements of the legs. These are commonly called diphasic dyskinesia because they occur during the transition from off to on and again during the transition from on to off. They are often associated with typical choreic dyskinesia at peak dose and seem to be related primarily to rapidly changing plasma levodopa levels.

Assessing Motor Fluctuations

The most important step in assessing motor fluctuations is to educate the patient about the characteristics of these fluctuations and to introduce a shared vocabulary for describing motor fluctuations. 'On' time refers to time when mobility is good and parkinsonian symptoms are minimized. 'Off' time refers to poor mobility. Dyskinesia refers to treatment-related involuntary movements, and it should be distinguished from rhythmic tremor.

The importance of discerning the pattern and timing of fluctuations and dyskinesia must be stressed. The use of 'on-off' diaries reinforces the patient's knowledge of fluctuations and helps the clinician determine the best intervention. Patients can complete 'on-off' diaries 2 days weekly for the 2 weeks before a scheduled appointment. One day should be a weekday, and the other should be a weekend day. Patients should make an hourly record, rating motor function at each waking time point as *Off*, *On*, or *On with dyskinesia* and record hours asleep. The time of meals and medications should also be noted on the diary form. Patients who are particularly protein sensitive can also be identified using these diaries. A typical 'on-off' diary is shown in Figure 6-2.

Treatment of Motor Fluctuations

Many PD experts now believe that the likelihood of developing motor response fluctuations can be reduced by the early use of dopamine agonist monotherapy.[12,13] Confirmation of this will require longer follow-up of patients randomized to these treatments in the clinical trials. However, dopamine agonist monotherapy may not be possible because of its increased expense and poorer tolerability. Moreover, since dopamine agonist monotherapy is not possible in patients with advanced PD, all patients require levodopa and nearly all patients will eventually develop significant motor fluctuations.

Treatment of wearing-off

For typical patients with mild-to-moderate disability and wearing-off, controlled-release carbidopa/levodopa (Sinemet® CR) may be useful because its administration results in a lower peak levodopa concentration and a longer duration of action. It is generally possible to reduce the frequency of dosing by about 30% and to improve symptom control by switching patients from standard to controlled-release carbidopa/levodopa. Controlled-release carbidopa/levodopa has a lower bioavailability than the standard preparation, so it is necessary to increase the total daily dose by 20% to 30% when making the conversion.[14] Patients who are used to the feeling of rapid improvement associated with standard carbidopa/levodopa (Sinemet®) may not like the delayed response experienced with controlled-release carbidopa/levodopa. Adding a small dose of standard carbidopa/levodopa or breaking the first controlled-release dose in half speeds absorption and helps alleviate this problem.

Another approach to patients with wearing-off, who often also have peak-dose dyskinesia, is dividing the dose of levodopa into smaller, more frequent doses. This is generally effective unless the incremental dose is too close to the threshold for reliable efficacy, at which point dose failures may become apparent.

For example, a patient taking carbidopa/levodopa 25/100 1.5 tablets at 7 AM, 2 PM, and 7 PM daily and experiencing early wearing-off can usually be managed by giving one tablet at 7 AM, 11 AM, 3 PM, and 0.5 to one tablet at 7 PM. While it is possible in most patients to stabilize wearing-off using increments of 0.5 to one tablet, some patients will require increments <0.5 tablets or between 0.5 and one tablet. In these more extreme cases, patients can prepare liquid levodopa, which can be titrated much more closely.

Liquid carbidopa/levodopa can be made by blending 10 tablets of 10/100 or 25/100 carbidopa/levodopa with 1 L of water. Powdered drink mix can be added to improve the taste of the solution (Table 6-2). Prepared in this way, liquid carbidopa/levodopa is stable at room temperature for up to 24 hours. The addition of ascorbic acid lengthens the stable period at room temperature to 72 hours, and the mixture can be refrigerated for up to 7 days.[15] Tight titration is possible with the resulting 1-mg levodopa/mL of the solution.

Liquid carbidopa/levodopa has a rapid onset of effect, but the low dose has a short duration of action, requiring hourly administration. The initial dose can be calculated by dividing the total daily dose of levodopa tablets by 13, and administering this fractional dose every hour between 7 AM and 7 PM. The first daily dose can be increased as needed, and many patients take a controlled-release carbidopa/levodopa at the end of the day (8 PM) to prevent nocturnal akinesia. It is important to stress to the patient that the initial dose calculation represents a best estimate of the required daily dose. Adjustments are likely and can be undertaken by telephone or office visit. In a double-blind, placebo-controlled study, administration of liquid carbidopa/levodopa reduced

Table 6-2: Preparation and Use of Liquid Carbidopa/Levodopa

Recipe for liquid carbidopa/levodopa 1 mg/mL Dose

- 10 tablets 25/100 standard carbidopa/levodopa in 1 liter of water

  or 5 tablets 25/100 standard carbidopa/levodopa in 500 cc water

- 500-mg vitamin C (optional)
- Powdered drink mix to taste

Mix all ingredients in standard blender. Store at room temperature up to 24 hours or in refrigerator up to 7 days.

Dosing

- Divide total daily dose by 13 to establish incremental dose.
- Add 20% incremental dose to first dose.
- Give incremental dose every hour from 7 AM to 7 PM.
- Give 25/100 or 50/200 controlled-release carbidopa/levodopa at bedtime for nocturnal akinesia.
- Adjust incremental dose based on 'on-off' diaries.

disability without increasing dyskinesia, despite a higher total daily dose of levodopa in the liquid-treatment arm.[16] In practice, liquid levodopa can be cumbersome for the patient. It is best reserved for younger patients with a very brittle response to medication.

Wearing-off can also be lessened by the addition of adjunctive medications, such as amantadine (Symmetrel®),[17] a catechol-o-methyltransferase (COMT) inhibitor,[18] MAO-B inhibitor, or a direct-acting dopamine agonist. The addition of an adjunctive agent in PD patients often makes it necessary to reduce the levodopa dosage. An evidence-based review found that entacapone (COMTan®) and rasagiline (Azilect®) are established as effective; pramipexole (Mirapex®), ropinirole (Requip®), and tolcapone (Tasmar®) are probably effective; and apomorphine subcutaneous injection and selegiline (Eldepryl®, Zelapar®) are possibly effective in reducing 'off' time in PD.[19] Although Eldepryl® and Zelapar® both feature the same active ingredient, selegiline, Eldepryl® and Zelapar® have different recommended dosages and different modes of administration. The recommended dosage of Eldepryl® is a divided dose of 10 mg/day, 5 mg to be taken at breakfast and 5 mg to be taken at dinner. The Eldepryl® dosage is swallowed, and the manufacturer recommends that it be taken at mealtimes. In contrast, Zelapar® is an orally disintegrating tablet (1.25 mg), which disintegrates within seconds after placement on the tongue and is rapidly absorbed. The target daily dose of Zelapar® is 2.5 mg. Table 6-3 describes the initial and target doses for these agents in the fluctuating PD patient. It should be noted that adding adjunctive medications for the treatment of motor fluctuations may require a reduction in the dose of other antiparkinsonian medications.

Although protein has a significant harmful effect on levodopa absorption from the gut and levodopa transport across the blood-brain barrier, most patients are not aware of the effect of protein ingestion on motor function. Thus, it is necessary to consider protein reduction only in those patients who have noticed such effects in themselves and whose diary review suggests a significant protein effect on 'off' time. A highly restricted diet that limits protein intake at breakfast and lunch to 7 g and allows liberal protein intake at the evening meal may substantially improve function in such protein-sensitive patients.[20] A balanced intake of 7 g of carbohydrate to 1 g of protein may also be useful. Consultation with a registered dietitian may be necessary to ensure that patients remain adequately nourished.

Table 6-3: Adjunctive Drugs for the Treatment of 'Wearing Off' Phenomenon in PD

Drug	Initial Dose	Target Dose
Amantadine (Symmetrel®)	100 mg daily	100 mg b.i.d. to t.i.d.
Entacapone (COMTan®)	200 mg with each levodopa dose	200 mg with each levopoda dose
Tolcapone (Tasmar®)	100 mg t.i.d.	100 to 200 mg t.i.d.
Bromocriptine (Parlodel®, Parlodel® SnapTabs®)	1.25 mg daily	5 to 15 mg t.i.d.
Pergolide* (Permax®)	0.125 mg t.i.d.	0.5 to 1 mg t.i.d.
Pramipexole (Mirapex®)	0.125 mg t.i.d.	0.5 to 1.5 mg t.i.d.
Ropinirole (Requip®)	0.25 mg t.i.d.	3 to 6 mg t.i.d
Rasagiline (Azilect®)	0.5 mg q.d.	0.5 to 1 mg q.d.
Selegiline (Eldepryl®)	10 mg q.d.	5 mg b.i.d.
Selegiline (Zelapar®)	1.25 mg q.d.	2.5 mg q.d.

*Pergolide (Permax®) and its generic products have been voluntarily withdrawn from the US market.

Treatment of 'on-off' motor fluctuations

'On-off' motor fluctuations are rare in PD, occurring in only about 10% of patients. The treatment of on-off is much more problematic than the treatment of wearing-off. Detailed pharmacologic studies in patients with 'on-off' syndrome show that the symptoms do not resolve with continuous intravenous levodopa infusion, suggesting that the mechanism of this motor fluctuation involves the actual dopamine receptor or downstream mechanisms.[4] The first step in treating 'on-off' syndrome is a detailed review of the medication response using 'on-off' diaries to help separate dose-related fluctuations that are likely to respond to interventions aimed at improving drug delivery to the brain. Adding a direct-acting dopamine agonist will help some patients. In addition, any patients with 'on-off' syndrome have advanced disease and are candidates for surgical intervention.

Treatment of Dyskinesia

The treatment of dyskinesia first depends on the accurate identification of the type of dyskinesia and its timing in relation to dopamine levels in the brain. Peak-dose dyskinesia is often not disabling, and patients often prefer its effects over the immobility that results if the drug dose is reduced. Dyskinesia tends to worsen over time. When it becomes disabling, the incremental dose of carbidopa/levodopa can be reduced and the interdose interval shortened as in the treatment of wearing-off. The addition of amantadine, 100 to 400 mg daily, may also reduce dyskinesia.[21] However, amantadine in these doses may produce confusion or hallucinations, so it should be used cautiously in the elderly and those with renal compromise, and not at all with significant cognitive impairment. Benzodiazepines may also be helpful. In severe cases, clozapine (Clozaril®) may be helpful.[22]

Dystonia in untreated PD may be treated with anticholinergic agents, such as trihexyphenidyl, 2 to 8 mg daily. In treated PD, end-of-dose dystonia usually responds to stabilization of the motor response as described in the treatment of wearing-off. The addition of a dopamine agonist to levodopa often improves the dystonia associated with wearing-off and with the early-morning 'off' period. Baclofen (Kemstro™, Lioresal®) 10 to 20 mg three times daily and at bedtime may also be useful.

Diphasic dyskinesias are difficult to treat. Optimizing drug delivery using the strategies outlined in the treatment of wearing-off, especially the addition of a direct-acting dopamine agonist, may be helpful. Depending on their ages and general health, these patients are usually candidates for surgical intervention (see Chapter 7).

Treatment-Resistant Symptoms: Freezing and Progressive Gait Disorder, Progressive Speech Disorders, and Swallowing Dysfunction

A far more troublesome and dangerous development in advanced PD is the emergence of treatment-resistant symptoms, such as freezing gait with falling, speech disorders, and swallowing dysfunction. These symptoms appear even as bradykinesia and rigidity, as assessed by repetitive limb movements, remain reasonably well controlled by dopaminergic drugs. Many investigators believe these more midline symptoms are related to lesions in nondopaminergic brain regions, and thus are refractory to dopamine receptor stimulation.[23,24]

Freezing and falling

Freezing refers to sudden arrests in movement. While freezing does occur in untreated PD, it is particularly disabling in patients with more advanced disease. The first sign of the development of freezing is start hesitation. The patient usually states that it takes a few seconds to initiate walking. Freezing gait may also be noticed immediately after turning. Terminal hesitation, slowing or freezing as one approaches an object such as a chair or counter, may begin at this time as well. Later, patients usually notice the tendency for shortened stride length or frank freezing in visually narrowed environments, such as when going through a doorway or entering an elevator. Turning usually becomes more difficult at this time. Eventually, patients may develop sudden arrests in foot movement when walking, as if the feet become stuck to the floor. Because upper body momentum continues, this type of freezing may precipitate a fall. Some patients may only freeze during 'off' periods, while others freeze even during the best daily 'on' time.

Falling is a late-onset symptom in PD. Falling during the first several years of a parkinsonian illness suggests another diagnosis, such as progressive supranuclear palsy or multiple system atrophy. In PD, falls are common, occurring in nearly half of patients with moderate or greater disability. A significant minority of patients (15%) fall at least once a week.[25] Complications of falls can be serious over a 10-year period, with nearly 30% of PD patients sustaining a hip fracture.[26] Falling is most common in elderly subjects and those with long-disease duration.

Potential contributors to falls in PD include gait bradykinesia, postural reflex impairment, freezing, and orthostatic hypotension. Cognitive dysfunction may make patients more careless about walking as well. Clinical studies have shown correlations between falls and patient age, disease duration, and postural reflex impairment, though not with other features of the illness.[25] Adjusting the antiparkinsonian drugs often does not lessen the frequency of falls.

Because patients generally do not fall in the physician's office, fall assessment relies primarily on patient history and physical assessment. The patient should be asked where the fall occurred. Many patients fall when pivoting in small areas, such as the bathroom, or when backing away from the refrigerator or kitchen counter. It is also useful to ask what the patient was doing when he or she fell. Fall-prone patients often fall when stooping, bending, or when carrying something. Tripping over throw rugs or thresholds is increased because PD patients do not lift their feet high enough to clear even low obstacles. When falling tends to occur in visually narrow environments, including doorways and elevators, freezing gait should be suspected. Patients who fall because of orthostatic hypotension usually experience symptoms of lightheadedness or presyncope before falling. The timing of falls may be helpful since falls during the 'off' period may respond to optimization of antiparkinsonian therapy. The office examination of falling PD patients should assess for concomitant neurologic and other dysfunction as well as pertinent parkinsonian signs such as postural reflexes and gait. Higher scores on the gait, posture, and pull-test items in the Unified Parkinson's Disease Rating Scale (UPDRS) predict falls in PD. The functional-reach test is a simple tool for assessing postural reflexes. The patient should stand with one shoulder close to the wall and the same arm outstretched with a closed fist. The patient reaches forward with the outstretched arm as far as possible without taking a step or falling over. The forward distance traveled by the closed fist is measured. A functional reach <6 inches is a significant risk factor for falls. Inability to stand on one leg for >10 seconds also may be a useful predictor of fall risk.[27]

The treatment of the progressive gait disorder of PD is difficult. Antiparkinsonian therapy should be optimized, particularly in patients who fall only during 'off' periods. Patients and family members should be educated about environmental contributors to freezing and falling, such as overcrowded living spaces, poor lighting, thick pile carpeting, and throw rugs. Environmental tricks can be used to facilitate walking, ie, playing marching music, placement of stripes on the carpet or flooring, or counting aloud or issuing marching orders during walking. Turning a conventional cane upside down and stepping over the handle often helps to initiate gait, as can a cane with a laser pointer affixed to shine a line perpendicular to the direction of travel.[28,29] Sometimes, a tactile stimulus (ie, kick or tap) to the foot or leg helps stepping. Support groups tend to be fertile fields for identification of these tricks. However, no trick consistently helps every patient. Physical therapy can be helpful at this stage of the illness.

Progressive speech disorders and swallowing dysfunction

Speech abnormalities occur frequently in PD, though they tend not to be prominent until moderate-to-advanced disease. PD patients produce speech with low volume and poor articulation. The timing of speech is often abnormal as well, with short rushes of speech and stuttering.[30] Dopaminergic stimulation does not reliably improve intelligibility, suggesting that nondopaminergic mechanisms contribute to these phenomena. Dysphagia affects up to 75% of patients with moderate-to-advanced disease.[31] Lung infections, related to aspiration and immobility, are among the most common causes of death in PD.[32] Detailed videofluoroscopic studies confirm the clinical impression that swallowing disorders respond poorly to dopaminergic therapy, suggesting that other nondopaminergic mechanisms also underlie this symptom. The assessment and treatment of speech disorders and swallowing dysfunction are examined in Chapter 9.

References

1.   Tolosa E, Valldeoriola F: Mid-stage parkinsonism with mild motor fluctuations. *Clin Neuropharmacol* 1994;17(suppl 2): S19-S31.

2.   Nutt JG, Holford NH: The response to levodopa in Parkinson's disease: imposing pharmacological law and order. *Ann Neurol* 1996;39: 561-573.

3.   Stocchi F, Bonamartini A, Vacca L, et al: Motor fluctuations in levodopa treatment: clinical pharmacology. *Eur Neurol* 1996;36 (suppl 1):38-42.

4.   Mouradian MM, Juncos JL, Fabbrini G, et al: Motor fluctuations in Parkinson's disease: central pathophysiological mechanisms, Part II. *Ann Neurol* 1988;24:372-378.

5.   Chapuis S, Ouchchane L, Metz O, et al: Impact of the motor complications of Parkinson's disease on the quality of life. *Mov Disord* 2005;20:224-230.

6.   Block G, Liss C, Reines S, et al: Comparison of immediate-release and controlled release carbidopa/levodopa in Parkinson's disease. A multicenter 5-year study. The CR First Study Group. *Eur Neurol* 1997;37:23-27.

7.   Mizuno Y, Kondo T, Mori H: Various aspects of motor fluctuations and their management in Parkinson's disease. *Neurology* 1994;44 (7 suppl 6):S29-S34.

8.   Pincus JH, Barry KM: Plasma levels of amino acids correlate with motor fluctuations in parkinsonism. *Arch Neurol* 1987;44:1006-1009.

9.   Mouradian MM, Juncos JL, Fabbrini G, et al: Motor fluctuations in Parkinson's disease: pathogenetic and therapeutic studies. *Ann Neurol* 1987;22:475-479.

10.   Antonini A, Schwarz J, Oertel WH, et al: Long-term changes of striatal dopamine D2 receptors in patients with Parkinson's disease: a study with positron emission tomography and [11C]raclopride. *Mov Disord* 1997;12:33-38.

11.   Fahn S: The spectrum of levodopa-induced dyskinesias. *Ann Neurol* 2000;47(4 suppl 1):S2-S11.

12.   A randomized controlled trial comparing pramipexole with levodopa in early Parkinson's disease: design and methods of the CALM-PD Study. Parkinson Study Group. *Clin Neuropharmacol* 2000;23:34-44.

13.   Rascol O, Brooks DJ, Korczyn AD, et al: A five-year study of the incidence of dyskinesia in patients with early Parkinson's disease who were treated with ropinirole or levodopa. 056 Study Group. *N Engl J Med* 2000;342:1484-1491.

14.   Manyam BV, Hare TA, Robbs R, et al: Evaluation of equivalent efficacy of sinemet and sinemet CR in patients with Parkinson's disease applying levodopa dosage conversion formula. *Clin Neuropharmacol* 1999;22:33-39.

15.   Pappert EJ, Buhrfiend C, Lipton JW, et al: Levodopa stability in solution: time course, environmental effects, and practical recommendations for clinical use. *Mov Disord* 1996;11:24-26.

16.   Pappert EJ, Goetz CG, Niederman F, et al: Liquid levodopa/carbidopa produces significant improvement in motor function without dyskinesia exacerbation. *Neurology* 1996;47:1493-1495.

17.   Shannon KM, Goetz CG, Carroll VS, et al: Amantadine and motor fluctuations in chronic Parkinson's disease. *Clin Neuropharmacol* 1987;10:522-526.

18.   Entacapone for Parkinson's disease. *Med Lett Drugs Ther* 2000; 42:7-8.

19.   Pahwa R, Factor SA, Lyons KE, et al: Practice Parameter: treatment of Parkinson disease with motor fluctuations and dyskinesia (an

evidence-based review): report of the Quality Standards Subcommittee of the American Academy of Neurology. *Neurology* 2006;66;983-995.

20. Pincus JH, Barry K: Protein redistribution diet restores motor function in patients with dopa-resistant "off" periods. *Neurology* 1988;38:481-483.

21. Verhagen Metman L, Del Dotto P, van den Munckhof P, et al: Amantadine as treatment for dyskinesias and motor fluctuations in Parkinson's disease. *Neurology* 1998;50:1323-1326.

22. Bennett JP Jr, Landow ER, Dietrich S, et al: Suppression of dyskinesias in advanced Parkinson's disease: moderate daily clozapine doses provide long-term dyskinesia reduction. *Mov Disord* 1994;9:409-414.

23. Bonnet AM, Loria Y, Saint-Hilaire MH, et al: Does long-term aggravation of Parkinson's disease result from nondopaminergic lesions? *Neurology* 1987;37:1539-1542.

24. Agid Y, Graybiel AM, Ruberg M, et al: The efficacy of levodopa treatment declines in the course of Parkinson's disease: do nondopaminergic lesions play a role? *Adv Neurol* 1990;53:83-100.

25. Koller WC, Glatt S, Vetere-Overfield B, et al: Falls and Parkinson's disease. *Clin Neuropharmacol* 1989;12:98-105.

26. Johnell O, Melton LJ III, Atkinson EJ, et al: Fracture risk in patients with parkinsonism: a population-based study in Olmsted County, Minnesota. *Age Ageing* 1992;21:32-38.

27. Jacobs JV, Horak FB, Tran VK, et al: Multiple balance tests improve the assessment of postural stability in subjects with Parkinson's disease. *J Neurol Neurosurg Psychiatry* 2006;77:322-326.

28. Dietz MA, Goetz CG, Stebbins GT: Evaluation of a modified inverted walking stick as a treatment for parkinsonian freezing episodes. *Mov Disord* 1990;5:243-247.

29. Kompoliti K, Goetz CG, Leurgans S, et al: "On" freezing in Parkinson's disease: resistance to visual cue walking devices. *Mov Disord* 2000;15:309-312.

30. Ramig LO, Countryman S, O'Brien C, et al: Intensive speech treatment for patients with Parkinson's disease: short- and long-term comparison of two techniques. *Neurology* 1996;47:1496-1504.

31. Johnston BT, Li Q, Castell JA, et al: Swallowing and esophageal function in Parkinson's disease. *Am J Gastroenterol* 1995;90: 1741-1746.

32. Wermuth L, Stenager EN, Stenager E, et al: Mortality in patients with Parkinson's disease. *Acta Neurol Scand* 1995;92:55-58.

Chapter 7

Surgical Management of Motor Dysfunction

Introduction and Historic Background
The need for and development of ablative surgical techniques

Since James Parkinson's pivotal monograph on paralysis agitans, clinicians have recognized that structural lesions in the motor pathways can improve the symptoms of parkinsonism. He described a 72-year-old parkinsonian man whose tremor and rigidity improved following an acute stroke.[1] This observation became the foundation for the development of ablative surgical techniques for the treatment of Parkinson's disease (PD) (Table 7-1). Early surgeons lesioned virtually every level of the motor system, including the spinal cord, cerebral cortex, and cerebral peduncle. Although tremor and rigidity often improved, weakness was an invariable accompaniment.[2] In 1952, Cooper inadvertently created the first pallidotomy in a PD patient when he ligated the anterior choroid artery, which he had damaged during a procedure for an unrelated condition.[3] This fortuitous calamity refocused surgical approaches on structures in the basal ganglia, especially the globus pallidus. In the 1960s, the favored target shifted to the ventrolateral thalamus after it became clear that thalamic lesions were more effective at reducing tremor. Surgical ablations soon became the favored approach for PD,[2,4,5] and an estimated 37,000 ablative procedures were performed on PD patients before 1969.[2] However, with the introduction of specific dopaminergic pharmacotherapy of PD, ablative surgery quickly became obsolete. However, as experience with chronic dopaminergic therapy grew, its limitations became obvious. Over the same period, advances in our understanding of basal ganglia physiology and improvements in stereotactic technique reawakened interest in the use of ablative lesions for patients with advanced PD who did not benefit from medical therapy.

The need for and development of restorative surgeries for PD

The failure of ablative surgical techniques and specific pharmacotherapy to affect the long-term course of PD has fueled the development of restorative surgical techniques that aim to repopulate areas of brain cell destruction. Grounded in substantial basic science literature that suggested human fetal cells had the potential to grow and develop in adult brains, the earliest restorative trials studied fetal substantia nigra cell transplantation into the striatum. Thrilling results using fetal tissue in animal models of PD have stimulated pilot studies in PD patients, and other techniques, including transplantation of other cell types, trophic factor infusions, and gene therapy, are under development. All restorative techniques remain highly experimental.

The popularity of surgical treatments among neurologists has waxed and waned. Nonetheless, patients continue to be acutely attracted to surgical treatments, which are made glamorous by their practitioners and the media.

Ablative Surgeries for Parkinson's Disease

Rationale and general principles

The basal ganglia are important in the selection and execution of complex programmed motor movements, which include initiation and maintenance of movement as well as prevention of unwanted or intrusive movements. This is accomplished by increasing or decreasing the inhibitory output of the globus pallidus on the thalamo-cortical pathways (see Chapter 3). In simple terms, in-

Table 7-1: Ablative Surgery for PD

Location	Symptoms Improved
Thalamus	Tremor, rigidity
Globus pallidus	Levodopa-induced dyskinesia, tremor, rigidity, bradykinesia
Subthalamic nucleus	Bradykinesia, tremor, rigidity, dyskinesia

creasing pallidal inhibitory activity brakes movement, while decreasing pallidal inhibitory activity facilitates movement. Several lines of scientific evidence suggest that in PD, inhibitory outflow from the globus pallidus to the thalamus dramatically increases. Activity of the subthalamic nucleus, which facilitates pallidal inhibitory outflow, also increases.[6] Because the increase in pallidal inhibitory outflow to the thalamus appears to be responsible for the paucity and slowness of movement in PD, it follows that attempts to decrease pallidal or subthalamic outflow may be successful in relieving this movement abnormality. The role of the thalamus in the production of parkinsonian tremor remains poorly understood. Micro-electrode recordings suggest that rhythmic discharges in the ventral intermediate nucleus underlie tremor in the contralateral limbs. These oscillations may originate in or be routed through the thalamus.[7] Thus, surgical lesions in the thalamus might obliterate or interrupt this rhythmic tremor generator.

Surgical PD treatment features two important concepts. The first is that, as in real estate, the most important aspects are 'location, location, location.' Thalamic procedures are effective for contralateral tremor and rigidity, but not brady-

Table 7-2: Need for Novel Approaches in PD

Levodopa-resistant symptoms
- Tremor
- Gait disorder
- Speech disorder

Long-term therapy complications
- Motor fluctuations
- Dyskinesia

kinesia. Procedures in the globus pallidus are dramatically effective for contralateral levodopa-induced dyskinesia, and less effective for contralateral bradykinesia, rigidity, and tremor. Subthalamic procedures are effective for contralateral bradykinesia, rigidity, tremor, and dyskinesia (Table 7-2).

The second concept is that there are two ways to reduce the activity of an overactive target: chemical or thermal destruction and high-frequency electric stimulation. Permanence is the most obvious drawback to outright destruction. Because unilateral lesion procedures influence contralateral symptoms, clinicians would expect them to have limited efficacy. Bilateral ablative lesions may cause cognitive impairment or severe speech abnormality, so these lesions are generally avoided in PD. However, the weight of evidence suggests that stimulation of deep-brain targets can safely be performed bilaterally.

Surgical procedures for PD should be performed at institutions where physicians are skilled in the diagnosis, medical management, and surgical treatment of PD. These procedures are performed with stereotactic localization using magnetic resonance imaging (MRI), computed tomography (CT), or both. The patient remains awake so physicians can make serial examinations for safety and efficacy. At many institutions, anatomic localization is confirmed by inserting a recording electrode into the deep-brain structures and recording neuronal firing patterns to make a physiologic map of the target. Physicians also stimulate the target to determine whether nearby structures, especially the motor and visual pathways, are at risk. Making a test lesion before the permanent lesion gives the surgeon final reassurance that vital structures are spared.[8] Limited studies exist of lesions produced using the gamma knife, and the results are somewhat mixed.[9,10] The major drawback of this technique is the inability to use neuronal recordings to physiologically map the target zone or to produce a test lesion in the region. Preliminary response rates may be lower than with other techniques, but the procedure is well tolerated and may be suited for patients who are poor surgical candidates.[9]

Deep-brain stimulators are implanted using stereotactic technique. The stimulating electrode has four stimulation sites near the tip. The pulse generator is implanted in the subclavicular chest wall. An external programming device allows changes in stimulation frequency, pulse width, and intensity and allows the choice of four stimulation sites. Patients can turn the device on and off using a hand-held magnet. The battery life ranges between 2 and 5 years, and is replaced in a simple surgical procedure. There have been reports of device failure or broken leads.

Thalamus: stereotactic thalamotomy and thalamic stimulation

Considering its importance in the history of PD surgery, the thalamus has become a relatively unpopular target for surgery in the modern age. Thalamotomy was popularized by Cooper,[3,11] who reported remarkable improvements in tremor and rigidity following lesions of the ventrolateral thalamic nucleus. Using electrophysiologic recording, Narabayashi and others determined that the ventralis intermedialis (VIM) nucleus was the most effective target.[12] Contralateral tremor was relieved in 70% to 90% of cases, but the procedure caused hypotonia in the limbs, and bradykinesia did not improve. Indeed, some clinicians believed bradykinesia was worse after surgery than before and that the operated side responded less well to levodopa. Since levodopa therapy was introduced, surgical series have been heavily weighted in favor of patients who failed medical management. However, reported success rates remain close to 90% with good maintenance of benefit at 2 years and 8% long-term morbidity.[13,14] Anecdotal reports exist that allege that thalamotomy prevents the subsequent development of dyskinesia on the side contralateral to surgery or that it lessens the rate of disease progression. Without controlled prospective studies, however, the veracity of these claims cannot be adequately evaluated.[12,15]

Using modern surgical techniques and well-selected patients, significant adverse effects are rare. Hand weakness, hemiparesis, speech disorders, abulia, and dyskinesia have been reported.[16-20] In addition, verbal deterioration was noted following left thalamotomy and visuospatial deterioration following right thalamotomy.[21] Bilateral surgery often causes balance impairment, dysarthria, dysphonia, and dysphagia and should not be performed.

The principal drawback to thalamotomy is its limited efficacy. Tremor is not a major source of disability in PD, and as the disease progresses, it is overshadowed by progressive bradykinesia and gait disorder. Medication again becomes the mainstay of therapy. Thalamotomy continues to be a viable treatment for patients with asymmetric drug-resistant tremor or patients with severe bilateral tremor scheduled for the implantation of a thalamic stimulator in the contralateral hemisphere. An argument can be made that thalamotomy has a levodopa-sparing effect in tremor-predominant patients, which may reduce the risk of levodopa-associated complications, and young tremor-predominant patients should have a thalamotomy.

However, until the role of levodopa therapy in the development of response fluctuations and disease progression is better defined, prudence dictates that thalamotomy be reserved for drug-resistant patients. Although there are no age restrictions, more limited benefit and increased surgical risk have been demonstrated in patients of advanced age or those with hypertension.

It was Benabid et al[22] who first observed that, in patients undergoing stereotactic thalamotomy, high-frequency electric stimulation of the thalamic target strikingly reduced contralateral tremor. Benabid et al also suggested electric stimulation of the thalamus might effectively control tremor. In Benabid and colleagues initial series, 88% of 91 PD patients had good control of tremor at 6 months, and long-term efficacy was demonstrated for up to 11 years. Multicenter studies, including those in which the raters were unaware of whether the stimulator was turned on or off, have confirmed moderate-to-marked benefit in about 85% of cases.[23,24] In a comparative study in which subjects were randomly selected to have thalamotomy or thalamic stimulation, stimulator-treated patients had better functional outcome and fewer adverse effects than did thalamotomy patients.[25] Adverse effects are generally well tolerated. Stimulation-related paresthesias are commonly reported and improve with reduction in stimulation intensity.[24] Ataxia, hemorrhage, and death have rarely been reported.[25] Like thalamotomy, thalamic stimulation does not improve important functional deficits such as gait disorder, so it has limited efficacy for patients with advanced disease.[26]

Globus Pallidus: Stereotactic Pallidotomy and Pallidal Stimulation

After falling into obscurity in the 1960s, a resurgence of interest in pallidotomy followed Laitinen's rather remarkable observation that 81% of PD patients had a favorable response to unilateral posteroventral pallidotomy.[27] More compelling was his observation that, unlike with thalamotomy, bradykinesia and tremor improved after pallidotomy.[27] Several authors have since reported 15% to 70% improvements in measures of tremor, rigidity and bradykinesia, particularly in the unmedicated or 'off' state in PD patients following unilateral posteroventral pallidotomy. Pallidotomy does not consistently improve measures of parkinsonism in the 'on' state, but does have a dramatic effect on troublesome levodopa-induced dyskinesias, which most authors report are dramatically reduced or eliminated.[28-41] In small series, the beneficial effects of pallidotomy have persisted up to 4 years, although certain functions, such as gait and midline bradykinesia, may begin to deteriorate after 12 months.[35] Physicians usually cannot reduce the patient's reliance on antiparkinsonian medications postoperatively. Several surgical adverse effects have been reported, including cortical or lobar intraparenchymal hemorrhage, ischemic stroke, hemianopsia, frontal lobe syndrome, hemiparesis, cognitive decline, and speech disorders.[29,30,41] Although most series report a ≤5% incidence of serious adverse effects, some centers have had serious complications in one third or more of patients.[41,42] Weight gain, sometimes massive, also has been reported at some centers.[30,43] Although the risks vary widely, most complications occur during the surgeon's initial experience with the procedure. Older patients may have a greater surgical risk and a less robust response to surgery. Although practiced by some surgeons,[44-46] simultaneous bilateral lesion placement carries a greater risk of morbidity. Even when the placement of the second lesion occurs more than 6 months after the placement of the first lesion, the benefits from the second lesion are less robust than the first, and morbidity is greater.[28] Therefore, the practice of bilateral contemporaneous or staged pallidotomy remains controversial. As experience with deep-brain stimulation has increased, the use of pallidotomy has all but disappeared.

Clinicians have studied pallidal stimulation as an alternative to stereotactic pallidotomy.[47-51] Pallidal stimulation can

113

be applied unilaterally for the same indications as stereotactic pallidotomy, can be used contralateral to pallidotomy,[49] or can be used bilaterally.[47,48,51] In an open-label, 6-month multicenter study of 41 PD subjects, of whom 38 received pallidal deep-brain stimulation, 36 with 6-month follow-up showed a 33% improvement in motor United Parkinson's Disease Rating Scale (UPDRS) score, a 36% improvement in activities of daily living, and an increase in good quality 'on' time from 28% at baseline to 64% of the waking day. Dyskinesia improved 67%. There was no significant decrease in dopaminergic medications. Common adverse events included hemorrhage (9.8%), increased dyskinesia (7.3%), dystonia (5%), and lead migration (5%). Dysarthria, seizure, infections, and other side effects occurred in about 2% of cases.[52] The safety record for the procedure is good. Most patients have side effects related to the stimulation, such as paresthesia. Seizures, transient weakness or speech and language disorders, and minor hemorrhages have been reported, but major morbidity is rare.[51,53] Some clinicians suggest that the expense of implanting, adjusting, and maintaining two stimulators is not justified by the limited benefits of bilateral pallidal stimulation.[54]

Subthalamic nucleus: subthalamotomy and subthalamic nucleus stimulation

Small lesions placed in the subthalamic nucleus of animals with experimental parkinsonism effectively reduced bradykinesia and tremor, but caused large-amplitude involuntary movements (ie, hemiballismus) in the contralateral limbs.[55] In a small series of PD patients, small lesions were less effective than thalamotomy in the control of tremor and rigidity; hemiballismus occurred in some patients.[56-58] The risk of hemiballismus has discouraged the use of stereotactic subthalamotomy in PD.

Bilateral subthalamic stimulation has emerged as the surgical procedure of choice for advanced PD. A multicenter study enrolled 102 subjects, 91 of whom had bilateral stimulators placed and 91 of whom had 6-month follow-up. There was about 50% improvement in motor UPDRS scores in the off-medication state and an increase in good quality 'on' time from 27% to 44% of the waking day. Subjects decreased their antiparkinsonian drugs by about 37%. Common (2% to 5% of cases) adverse effects included infection, hemorrhage, seizures, increased dyskinesia, improper lead placement, lead breakage or migration, and device infection. Additional side effects included dysarthria, headache, paresthesia, confusion, paralysis, pulmonary embolus, seroma, and skin erosion.[52] Other studies show similar improvements in PD severity in 'off' time, dyskinesia prevalence and severity, ability to reduce dopaminergic medications, and similar adverse effects.[53] Gait symptoms, including troublesome gait freezing, may be responsive to the treatment.[59] Subthalamic nucleus deep-brain stimulation leads to significant improvement in quality of life that is sustained for at least 2 years.[60] The consistently reduced need for levodopa after subthalamic nucleus stimulation is the most compelling evidence in favor of its superiority among functional neurosurgeries for the symptomatic treatment of PD.

Restorative Surgeries for PD

Neural transplantation in PD

The concept that transplantation of dopaminergic neurons might reverse the biochemical and functional deficits in PD has strong support in the literature. PD is an ideal candidate disease for successful transplantation. A well-understood and localized neurodegenerative process with a single neurotransmitter deficit accounts for the major motor manifestations of the illness. The target tissue for the transplant is spared the degenerative process and is a well-circumscribed brain region of reasonable size. Human fetal substantia nigra cells transplanted into the striata of animals with experimental parkinsonism survive, mature, establish functional cell-to-cell interactions, release dopamine, and reverse the behavioral abnormalities characteristic of the experimental condition.[61-63]

For transplantation to be a valuable therapeutic intervention, the following conditions must be met: the cells to be transplanted must be readily available and must be capable of surviving in large numbers, developing into organotypic dopaminergic neurons and establishing normal cell-to-cell interconnections; rejection potential must be low or anti-rejection strategies must be well tolerated and effective; the transplantation procedure must be safe; the procedure must allow distribution of the cells in a density that will maximize reinnervation of the denervated striatum; and well-controlled clinical trials must establish the efficacy and safety of the procedure.

Several cell types have been considered for use in PD, including adrenal medullary cells, encapsulated pheochromocytoma cells, retinal cells, human fetal substantia nigra cells, carotid body glomus cells, and neuronal progenitor (ie, stem) cells. The first human studies of neural transplantation used adrenal medullary cells. Removed from the steroid influence of the overlying adrenal cortex, adrenal medullary cells assume a morphology like neurons, form rudimentary processes, and increase dopamine synthesis. When transplanted into the brains of animals with experimental parkinsonism, there is some integration, but little fiber formation and little or no striatal innervation. However, behavioral manifestations of the experimental parkinsonism may be improved.[64]

In 1982 and 1983, two patients had stereotactic implantation of adrenal medullary tissue into the right caudate nucleus. Both patients had modest and short-lived improvements in contralateral rigidity and mobility.[65] Later, two patients received stereotactic implants of adrenal medullary tissue into the putamen. Modest benefits also were reported in these patients.[66] Shortly thereafter, a bold report suggested that open implantation of adrenal medullary autografts into a cavity created in the right caudate nucleus produced dramatic improvements in rigidity, tremor, and bradykinesia in PD patients.[67] Based on these anecdotal reports, several centers began performing the technique. Patient selection, operative technique, and pre- and post-operative assessments varied from institution to institution, limiting the generalization of experimental findings. In a literature review of 248 cases performed at more than 30 clinical centers, 66% of patients had modest improvements at 6 months. However, the rate of major morbidity and death was 12.5%.[68] Data collected prospectively on a series of 61 patients operated on at several sites confirmed that the benefits of surgery were modest and improvements were not sustained for 2 years. Postoperative morbidity, particularly psychiatric and pulmonary, was common.[69] Autopsy studies in 13 cases primarily showed gliosis and inflammation.[68] Dopaminergic cells were seen in only two cases.[70,71] The transient and modest improvements were thought by many to represent either a subacute injury response or some type of trophic influence. The adrenal medullary transplant procedure was eventually abandoned.

From this experience, clinicians realized we were unlikely to benefit from small clinical trials of neural transplantation in PD and that clinical evaluation protocols were essential to standardize patient selection and efficacy evaluations. Committees of investigators devised the Core Assessment Program for Intracerebral Transplantations (CAPIT) and, later, the Core Assessment Program for Surgical Interventional Therapies in Parkinson's Disease (CAPSIT-PD). Such tools have become routine in the preoperative selection and assessment of surgical patients and in their postoperative assessment.[72,73] The CAPIT and CAPSIT-PD protocols include tools for standardizing assessments of motor severity and disability, and assessing the patient's response to levodopa.

Human fetal substantia nigra transplantation into the striatum has solid support in the literature. Considerable animal data are available from which to extrapolate optimal transplantation techniques regarding selection of donor tissue, donor age, amount of tissue implanted, preparation of tissue, and targeted sites. Despite the animal experience, early human trials of human fetal substantia nigra transplants into the striatum were often flawed because physicians used donor cells of the wrong age, implanted an inadequate number of cells, or implanted them into the wrong regions of the host brain, and followed other methods demonstrated to be ineffective in animal models.[74,75] Equally sobering is the realization that in some patients who have been thought to respond clinically to human fetal transplants, methods were used that basic research suggests are unlikely to produce viable integrated grafts. This latter observation raises the specter of investigator bias, placebo effect, or nonspecific effect of surgery, and underscores the need for controlled clinical trials.

The most promising of the small, open-label pilot trials of fetal cell transplantation used fetal cells from the ventral mesencephalon of six to eight donor fetuses of 5 to 9 weeks' postconception age. These were stereotactically implanted into the postcommissural putamen bilaterally in staged surgeries. Patients were immunosuppressed with cyclosporine (Gengraf®, Neoral®, Sandimmune®) perioperatively and for 6 months postoperatively. Postoperatively, patients followed a course suggesting a transplant effect. Improvements were delayed and gradually progressive. Patients had reduced duration and severity of daily 'off' time with improvements in 'on' time and reduced dependence on antiparkinsonian medications.[76] Positron emission tomography (PET) studies confirmed a progressive postoperative increase in fluorodopa uptake. Most importantly, autopsy studies in two patients demonstrated viable dopaminergic neurons with large numbers of fibers crossing the graft-host interface and innervating the host brain.[77,78] The graft showed no evidence of the neurodegenerative process of PD. Although these preliminary results are encouraging, parkinsonian symptoms were only partially relieved by the procedure and only 5% to 10% of grafted neurons survived transplantation.[77,78] There have been two prospective, randomized, double-blind sham surgery-controlled clinical trials of human fetal striatal transplantation in PD. One study randomly assigned 40 subjects with advanced PD to bilateral implantation of fetal substantia nigra from a single embryo per side or to a sham procedure. There was no significant improvement in the primary outcome measure, although younger transplanted subjects showed a significant improvement in measures of motor severity.[79] A second study randomly assigned 34 subjects with advanced PD to bilateral implantation of fetal substantia nigra tissue from one embryo per side, four embryos per side, or to a sham procedure. At 2 years, there was no significant improvement in the primary outcome variable, though more mildly affected subjects did show a treatment effect.[80] In both studies, there were improvements in PET scan measures of dopaminergic activity in the striatum. However, because of the lackluster clinical benefits, these studies have effectively chilled research into this potential therapeutic strategy.

These human trials are an important step in establishing the potential of neural transplantation in PD. They demonstrate that, in carefully selected patients, an experienced team can safely transplant immature dopaminergic cells that survive, integrate into the host brain, and produce clinical effects. In the wrong hands, the outcome of transplantation ranges from ineffective to deadly. There have been two reported fatalities associated with inept fetal tissue dissection or operative technique, one caused by acute obstruction of the ventricular system and the other by development of an intraparenchymal cyst.[81,82] Limitless questions remain on how best to restore dopaminergic circuitry in the human brain. Some questions, such as optimal donor age, volume of cells, graft location, and methods of enhancing cell survival, can be answered in part in the animal laboratory. However, only controlled clinical trials will provide a believable answer about the clinical utility of methods developed in the animal laboratory.

Even in the best hands, however, it is unrealistic to expect that human fetal transplantation will ever become a part of the treatment regimen for PD. The technical expertise for tissue dissection and implantation is beyond the capabilities of all but the most highly specialized centers. Tissue procurement is difficult, and social and ethical obstacles exist to the large-scale use of fetal tissue. Development of a renewable source of pluripotent human cells (ie, genetically modified established cell lines, autologous cells, stem cells) and enhancements of techniques that dramatically increase cell survival and improve the distribution of cells into the denervated brain would make the procedure more viable. Work with other cell sources, such as neuronal progenitor (stem) cells, looks promising in the laboratory,[83,84] but has not yet reached the clinical trial stage.

One cell-based therapy that is in clinical testing is Spheramine®. This technology employs retinal pigment epithelial cells attached to microcarriers. In an open-label pilot study in six subjects with advanced PD, MRI-guided stereotactic implantation of 325,000 cells into the postcommissural putamen contralateral to the most affected side was associated with improvements in 'off' motor UPDRS scores. There was even some improvement on the ipsilateral side.[85] These findings are being tested in an ongoing prospective double-blind, sham-surgery, controlled clinical trial.

Gene Therapy

Laboratory studies of gene therapy suggest the potential usefulness of these techniques for PD.[86] Gene therapy techniques may be used to introduce a gene product that may protect against neurodegeneration or one that controls the synthesis of dopamine.

Two basic types of gene therapy exist. In ex vivo gene therapy, cells are modified in vitro and then transplanted into the organism. In in vivo gene therapy, genes are directly transferred to target tissues using viral vectors (Figure 7-1).

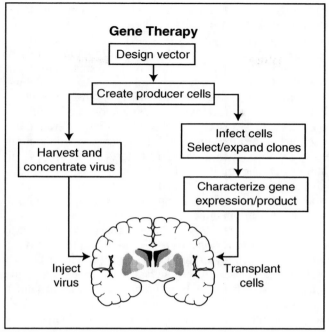

Gene Therapy

Design vector

Create producer cells

Infect cells
Select/expand clones

Harvest and
concentrate virus

Characterize gene
expression/product

Inject
virus

Transplant
cells

Figure 7-1: Ex vivo and in vivo gene therapy for Parkinson's disease (PD): A viral or other vector is selected. Cells containing the vector are created in the laboratory. The in vivo technique collects and concentrates the virus expressing the desired gene, and the virus is injected into the brain parenchyma. In the ex vivo technique, transfected cells are transplanted into the brain after the expression of the desired genetic product is confirmed.

The main advantage of ex vivo gene therapy is that clinicians can examine the cells to see if the transgene is functioning before transplantation. The transgene can be introduced into the cells by plasmid or retroviral vectors. Clinicians can make transfected cells that produce neurotrophic factors, such as brain-derived neurotrophic factor (BDNF), glial cell-derived neurotrophic factor (GDNF), or ciliary neurotrophic factor (CNTF). Alternatively, cells can be made to produce enzymes such as tyrosine hydroxylase, the rate-limiting enzyme for dopamine formation. Schwann cells, astrocytes, and stem cells have been studied for their potential to express transgenes and to survive transplantation without excessive immunogenicity or mitotic potential. A theoretic advantage exists in using neural cells because they have the potential to make afferent and efferent connections within the host brain. However, even nonneural cells show promise in animal models of PD. In several studies, transplantation of cells engineered to express neurotrophic factors reduced the extent of neurodegeneration in experimental parkinsonism or increased the central production of dopamine.[87-89]

In vivo gene transfer has advantages over ex vivo procedures because host nervous system cells should have a greater capacity than other cells to synthesize, package, and secrete the desired products and because there is no interference with normal brain architecture by transplanted cells. Clinicians have studied several viral vectors including herpes simplex type I, adenovirus, adeno-associated virus vector, retrovirus, and lentivirus.[90-93]

A number of gene therapy clinical trials are underway. A preliminary open-label study of unilateral subthalamic nucleus delivery of the glutamic acid decarboxylase gene by a nonpathogenic adeno-associated viral vector in 12 subjects with advanced PD showed contralateral improvements in motor disease severity and salutary changes in fluorodeoxyglucose imaging studies. The goal of this gene therapy technique is to increase inhibitory neurotransmitter synthesis in the subthalamic nucleus to decrease its overactivity.[94] Early clinical trials with viral vector delivery of the aromatic acid decarboxylase gene and with the gene for neurturin, a neurotrophin in the glial-derived neurotrophic factor family of ligands, are also in progress.

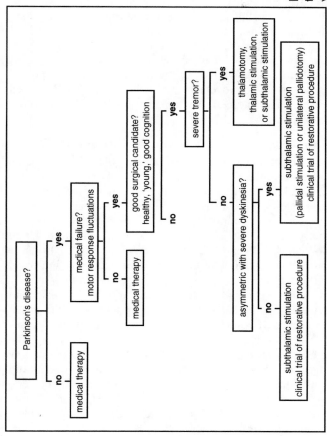

Figure 7-2: Decision tree for surgical intervention in PD.

Parkinson's disease?

no → medical therapy

yes → medical failure? motor response fluctuations

no → medical therapy

yes → good surgical candidate? healthy, 'young,' good cognition

no

yes → severe tremor?

yes → thalamotomy, thalamic stimulation, or subthalamic stimulation

no → asymmetric with severe dyskinesia?

yes → subthalamic stimulation (pallidal stimulation or unilateral pallidotomy) clinical trial of restorative procedure

no → subthalamic stimulation clinical trial of restorative procedure

7

Other Surgical Treatments

Intraparenchymal injections of neurotrophic factors have been successful in preventing neurodegeneration in animal models of parkinsonism.[95,96] However, an early human trial has failed to demonstrate any benefits of intraventricular injections of GDNF. In the autopsy of a patient who received intraventricular GDNF injections, the brain showed changes of advanced PD. There was an intense rim of tyrosine hydroxylase and dopamine transporter immunoreactivity along the medial rim of the caudate nucleus, the significance of which is unknown.[97] A randomized, double-blind study of bilateral putaminal delivery of GDNF or placebo using an implanted pump in 34 subjects with advanced PD showed no significant improvement at 6 months in the GDNF-treated group.[98] The future of such human trials of GDNF and other trophic factors is uncertain.

The Role of Surgery in the Treatment of PD

Current estimates are that 2% to 10% of PD patients might be suitable candidates for approved surgical procedures, suggesting that surgical treatments have a minor presence in the overall treatment of PD. They offer hope for selected patients with PD who have had robust benefit from conventional medical treatment, but who have failed secondarily because of motor response fluctuations or other complications of therapy. Elderly patients and those with significant cognitive impairments generally do poorly with these techniques. Patients with atypical parkinsonism have repeatedly been shown to fare poorly. A multitude of unanswered questions about surgical techniques remain, particularly in regard to transplantation and gene therapy. The medical community is grappling with questions about how rigorous clinical trials should be of surgical treatments and particularly about the need for surgical trials with placebo or sham-surgery control groups.[99] A decision tree (Figure 7-2) outlines how disease criteria should be used to select patients for surgical intervention.

References

1. Parkinson J: *An Essay on the Shaking Palsy.* London, Whittingham and Rowland, 1817.

2. Speelman JD, Bosch DA: Resurgence of functional neurosurgery for Parkinson's disease: a historical perspective. *Mov Disord* 1998;13:582-588.

3. Cooper IS: Surgical treatment of parkinsonism. *Br Med J* 1961;1: 1248-1249.

4. Guridi J, Lozano AM: A brief history of pallidotomy. *Neurosurgery* 1997;41:1169-1180; discussion 1180-1183.

5. Koller WC, Pahwa R, Lyons KE, et al: Surgical treatment of Parkinson's disease. *J Neurol Sci* 1999;167:1-10.

6. Hallett M: Physiology of basal ganglia disorders: an overview. *Can J Neurol Sci* 1993;20:177-183.

7. Lenz FA, Vitek JL, DeLong MR: Role of the thalamus in parkinsonian tremor: evidence from studies in patients and primate models. *Stereotact Funct Neurosurg* 1993;60:94-103.

8. Vitek JL, Bakay RA, Hashimoto T, et al: Microelectrode-guided pallidotomy: technical approach and its application in medically intractable Parkinson's disease. *J Neurosurg* 1998;88: 1027-1043.

9. Duma CM, Jacques D, Kopyov OV: The treatment of movement disorders using gamma knife stereotactic radiosurgery. *Neurosurg Clin N Am* 1999;10:379-389.

10. Friedman DP, Goldman HW, Flanders AE, et al: Stereotactic radiosurgical pallidotomy and thalamotomy with the gamma knife: MR imaging findings with clinical correlation—preliminary experience. *Radiology* 1999;212:143-150.

11. Cooper IS: Surgical treatment of parkinsonism. *Annu Rev Med* 1965;16:309-330.

12. Narabayashi H, Maeda T, Yokochi F: Long-term follow-up study of nucleus ventralis intermedius and ventrolateralis thalamotomy using a microelectrode technique in parkinsonism. *Appl Neurophysiol* 1987;50:330-337.

13. Tasker RR, Siqueira J, Hawrylyshyn P, et al: What happened to VIM thalamotomy for Parkinson's disease? *Appl Neurophysiol* 1983;46:68-83.

7

14. Wester K, Hauglie-Hanssen E: Stereotaxic thalamotomy—experiences from the levodopa era. *J Neurol Neurosurg Psychiatry* 1990;53:427-430.

15. Matsumoto K, Asano T, Baba T, et al: Long-term follow-up results of bilateral thalamotomy for parkinsonism. *Appl Neurophysiol* 1976;39:257-260.

16. Brophy BP, Kimber TJ, Thompson PD: Thalamotomy for parkinsonian tremor. *Stereotact Funct Neurosurg* 1997;69:1-4.

17. Fox MW, Ahlskog JE, Kelly PJ: Stereotactic ventrolateralis thalamotomy for medically refractory tremor in post-levodopa era Parkinson's disease patients. *J Neurosurg* 1991;75:723-730.

18. Goodman SH, Wilkinson S, Overman J, et al: Lesion volume and clinical outcome in stereotactic pallidotomy and thalamotomy. *Stereotact Funct Neurosurg* 1998;71:164-172.

19. Jankovic J, Cardoso F, Grossman RG, et al: Outcome after stereotactic thalamotomy for parkinsonian, essential, and other types of tremor. *Neurosurgery* 1995;37:680-687.

20. Keller TM, Tcheng TK, Burkhard PR, et al: Stereotactically guided thalamotomy for treatment of parkinsonian tremor isolated to the lower extremity. Case report. *J Neurosurg* 1998;89:314-316.

21. Wester K, Hugdahl K: Thalamotomy and thalamic stimulation: effects on cognition. *Stereotact Funct Neurosurg* 1997;69 (1-4 pt 2): 80-85.

22. Benabid AL, Benazzouz A, Hoffmann D, et al: Long-term electrical inhibition of deep brain targets in movement disorders. *Mov Disord* 1998;13(suppl 3):119-125.

23. Limousin P, Speelman JD, Gielen F, et al: Multicentre European study of thalamic stimulation in parkinsonian and essential tremor. *J Neurol Neurosurg Psychiatry* 1999;66:289-296.

24. Koller W, Pahwa R, Busenbark K, et al: High-frequency unilateral thalamic stimulation in the treatment of essential and parkinsonian tremor. *Ann Neurol* 1997;42:292-299.

25. Schuurman PR, Bosch DA, Bossuyt PM, et al: A comparison of continuous thalamic stimulation and thalamotomy for suppression of severe tremor. *N Engl J Med* 2000;342:461-468.

26. Defebvre LJ, Blatt JL, Blond SC, et al: Effect of long-term stimulation of the ventral intermediate thalamic nucleus on gait in Parkinson's disease. *Adv Neurol* 1999;80:627-630.

27. Laitinen LV: Pallidotomy for Parkinson's disease. *Neurosurg Clin N Am* 1995;6:105-112.

28. Alterman RL, Kelly PJ: Pallidotomy technique and results: the New York University experience. *Neurosurg Clin N Am* 1998; 9:337-343.

29. Baron MS, Vitek JL, Bakay RA, et al: Treatment of advanced Parkinson's disease by posterior GPi pallidotomy: 1-year results of a pilot study. *Ann Neurol* 1996;40:355-366.

30. Dalvi A, Winfield L, Yu Q, et al: Stereotactic posteroventral pallidotomy: clinical methods and results at 1-year follow up. *Mov Disord* 1999;14:256-261.

31. de Bie RM, de Haan RJ, Nijssen PC, et al: Unilateral pallidotomy in Parkinson's disease: a randomised, single-blind, multicentre trial. *Lancet* 1999;354:1665-1669.

32. Desaloms JM, Krauss JK, Lai EC, et al: Posteroventral medial pallidotomy for treatment of Parkinson's disease: preoperative magnetic resonance imaging features and clinical outcome. *J Neurosurg* 1998;89:194-199.

33. Dogali M, Fazzini E, Kolodny E, et al: Stereotactic ventral pallidotomy for Parkinson's disease. *Neurology* 1995;45:753-761.

34. Eller TW, Dan DA: Stereotactic pallidotomy for treatment of Parkinson's disease (published erratum appears in *AORN J* 1997; 66:224). *AORN J* 1997;65:903-904, 907-916; quiz 917-920.

35. Fazzini E, Dogali M, Sterio D, et al: Stereotactic pallidotomy for Parkinson's disease: a long-term follow-up of unilateral pallidotomy. *Neurology* 1997;48:1273-1277.

36. Hailey D, Harstall C: Posteroventral pallidotomy for Parkinson's disease: assessment and policy on a technology in transition. *Health Policy* 1998;43:55-64.

37. Kondziolka D, Bonaroti E, Baser S, et al: Outcomes after stereotactically guided pallidotomy for advanced Parkinson's disease. *J Neurosurg* 1999;90:197-202.

38. Kumar R, Lozano AM, Montgomery E, et al: Pallidotomy and deep brain stimulation of the pallidum and subthalamic nucleus in advanced Parkinson's disease. *Mov Disord* 1998;13:73-82.

39. Lozano AM, Lang AE, Galvez-Jimenez N, et al: Effect of GPi pallidotomy on motor function in Parkinson's disease. *Lancet* 1995;346:1383-1387.

40.   Samii A, Turnbull IM, Kishore A, et al: Reassessment of unilateral pallidotomy in Parkinson's disease. A 2-year follow-up study (see comments). *Brain* 1999;122(pt 3):417-425.

41.   Shannon KM, Penn RD, Kroin JS, et al: Stereotactic pallidotomy for the treatment of Parkinson's disease. Efficacy and adverse effects at 6 months in 26 patients. *Neurology* 1998;50:434-438.

42.   Sutton JP, Couldwell W, Lew MF, et al: Ventroposterior medial pallidotomy in patients with advanced Parkinson's disease. *Neurosurgery* 1995;36:1112-1117.

43.   Ondo WG, Ben-Aire L, Jankovic J, et al: Weight gain following unilateral pallidotomy in Parkinson's disease. *Acta Neurol Scand* 2000;101:79-84.

44.   Ghika J, Ghika-Schmid F, Fankhauser H, et al: Bilateral contemporaneous posteroventral pallidotomy for the treatment of Parkinson's disease: neuropsychological and neurological side effects. Report of four cases and review of the literature. *J Neurosurg* 1999;91:313-321.

45.   Siegel KL, Metman LV: Effects of bilateral posteroventral pallidotomy on gait of subjects with Parkinson disease. *Arch Neurol* 2000;57:198-204.

46.   Schuurman PR, de Bie RM, Speelman JD, et al: Posteroventral pallidotomy in movement disorders. *Acta Neurochir Suppl (Wien)* 1997;68:14-17.

47.   Ardouin C, Pillon B, Peiffer E, et al: Bilateral subthalamic or pallidal stimulation for Parkinson's disease affects neither memory nor executive functions: a consecutive series of 62 patients. *Ann Neurol* 1999;46:217-223.

48.   Volkmann J, Sturm V, Weiss P, et al: Bilateral high-frequency stimulation of the internal globus pallidus in advanced Parkinson's disease. *Ann Neurol* 1998;44:953-961.

49.   Galvez-Jimenez N, Lozano A, Tasker R, et al: Pallidal stimulation in Parkinson's disease patients with a prior unilateral pallidotomy. *Can J Neurol Sci* 1998;25:300-305.

50.   Gross C, Rougier A, Guehl D, et al: High-frequency stimulation of the globus pallidus internalis in Parkinson's disease: a study of seven cases. *J Neurosurg* 1997;87:491-498.

51.   Pahwa R, Wilkinson S, Smith D, et al: High-frequency stimulation of the globus pallidus for the treatment of Parkinson's disease. *Neurology* 1997;49:249-253.

52.   Deep-Brain Stimulation for Parkinson's Disease Study Group: Deep-brain stimulation of the subthalamic nucleus or the pars interna of the globus pallidus in Parkinson's disease. *N Engl J Med* 2001;345:956-963.

53.   Pahwa R, Factor SA, Lyons KE, et al: Practice Parameter: treatment of Parkinson disease with motor fluctuations and dyskinesia (an evidence-based review): report of the Quality Standards Subcommittee of the American Academy of Neurology. *Neurology* 2006;66:983-985.

54.   Tronnier VM, Fogel W, Kronenbuerger M, et al: Pallidal stimulation: an alternative to pallidotomy? *J Neurosurg* 1997;87: 700-705.

55.   Guridi J, Herrero MT, Luquin MR, et al: Subthalamotomy in parkinsonian monkeys. Behavioural and biochemical analysis. *Brain* 1996;119(pt 5):1717-1727.

56.   Andy OJ, Jurko MF, Sias FR Jr: Subthalamotomy in treatment of Parkinsonian tremor. *J Neurosurg* 1963;20:860-870.

57.   Gill SS, Heywood P: Bilateral dorsolateral subthalamotomy for advanced Parkinson's disease. *Lancet* 1997;350:1224.

58.   Hullay J: Subthalamotomy in Parkinson's disease. Analysis of responses to electrostimulation. *Acta Med Acad Sci Hung* 1971; 28:57-68.

59.   Yokoyama T, Sugiyama K, Nishizawa S, et al: Subthalamic nucleus stimulation for gait disturbance in Parkinson's disease. *Neurosurgery* 1999;45:41-49.

60.   Lezcano E, Gomez-Esteban JC, Zarranz JS, et al: Improvement in quality of life in patients with advanced Parkinson's disease following bilateral deep-brain stimulation in subthalamic nucleus. *Eur J Neurol* 2004;11:451-454.

61.   Widner H: The case for neural tissue transplantation as a treatment for Parkinson's disease. *Adv Neurol* 1999;80:641-649.

62.   Taylor JR, Elsworth JD, Roth RH, et al: Grafting of fetal substantia nigra to striatum reverses behavioral deficits induced by MPTP in primates: a comparison with other types of grafts as controls. *Exp Brain Res* 1991;85:335-348.

63.   Nikkhah G, Rosenthal C, Falkenstein G, et al: Dopaminergic graft-induced long-term recovery of complex sensorimotor behaviors in a rat model of Parkinson's disease. *Zentralbl Neurochir* 1998;59:97-103.

64.   Freed WJ, Morhisa M, Spoor HE, et al: Transplanted adrenal chromaffin cells in rat brain reduce lesion-induced rotational behavior. *Nature* 1981;292:351-352.

65.   Backlund EO, Granberg PO, Hamberger B, et al: Transplantation of adrenal medullary tissue to striatum in parkinsonism. First clinical trials. *J Neurosurg* 1985;62:169-173.

66.   Lindvall O, Backlund EO, Farde L, et al: Transplantation in Parkinson's disease: two cases of adrenal medullary grafts to the putamen. *Ann Neurol* 1987;22:457-468.

67.   Madrazo I, Drucker-Colin R, Diaz V, et al: Open microsurgical autograft of adrenal medulla to the right caudate nucleus in two patients with intractable Parkinson's disease. *N Engl J Med* 1987;316: 831-834.

68.   Shannon K, Goetz C: Transplantation of adrenal medullary tissue to brain in Parkinson's disease. In: Koller WC, Paulson G, eds: *Therapy of Parkinson's Disease*, 2nd ed. New York, NY, Marcel Dekker, 1995, pp 423-434.

69.   Goetz CG, Stebbins GT, Klawans HL, et al: United Parkinson Foundation Neurotransplantation Registry on adrenal medullary transplants: presurgical, and 1- and 2-year follow-up. *Neurology* 1991;41:1719-1722.

70.   Hirsch EC, Duyckaerts C, Javoy-Agid F, et al: Does adrenal graft enhance recovery of dopaminergic neurons in Parkinson's disease? *Ann Neurol* 1990;27:676-682.

71.   Kordower JH, Cochran E, Penn RD, et al: Putative chromaffin cell survival and enhanced host-derived TH-fiber innervation following a functional adrenal medulla autograft for Parkinson's disease. *Ann Neurol* 1991;29:405-412.

72.   Langston JW, Widner H, Goetz CG, et al: Core assessment program for intracerebral transplantations (CAPIT). *Mov Disord* 1992;7:2-13.

73.   Defer GL, Widner H, Marie RM, et al: Core Assessment program for surgical interventional therapies in Parkinson's disease (CAPSIT-PD). *Mov Disord* 1999;14:472-584.

74.   Freeman TB, Sanberg PR, Nauert GM, et al: The influence of donor age on the survival of solid and suspension intraparenchymal human embryonic nigral grafts. *Cell Transplant* 1995;4:141-154.

75.   Freeman TB, Sanberg PR, Isacson O: Development of the human striatum: implications for fetal striatal transplantation in

the treatment of Huntington's disease. *Cell Transplant* 1995;4: 539-545.

76.   Freeman TB, Olanow CW, Hauser RA, et al: Bilateral fetal nigral transplantation into the postcommissural putamen in Parkinson's disease. *Ann Neurol* 1995;38:379-388.

77.   Kordower JH, Freeman TB, Snow BJ, et al: Neuropathological evidence of graft survival and striatal reinnervation after the transplantation of fetal mesencephalic tissue in a patient with Parkinson's disease. *N Engl J Med* 1995;332:1118-1124.

78.   Kordower JH, Freeman TB, Chen EY, et al: Fetal nigral grafts survive and mediate clinical benefit in a patient with Parkinson's disease. *Mov Disord* 1998;13:383-393.

79.   Freed CR, Greene PE, Breeze RE, et al: Transplantation of embryonic dopamine neurons for severe Parkinson's disease. *N Engl J Med* 2001;344:710-719.

80.   Olanow CW, Goetz CG, Kordower JH, et al: A double-blind controlled trial of bilateral nigral transplantation in Parkinson's disease. *Ann Neurol* 2003;54:403-414.

81.   Mamelak AN, Eggerding FA, Oh DS, et al: Fatal cyst formation after fetal mesencephalic allograft transplant for Parkinson's disease. *J Neurosurg* 1998;89:592-598.

82.   Folkerth RD, Durso R: Survival and proliferation of nonneural tissues, with obstruction of cerebral ventricles, in a parkinsonian patient treated with fetal allografts. *Neurology* 1996;46:1219-1225.

83.   Baetge EE: Neural stem cells for CNS transplantation. *Ann NY Acad Sci* 1993;695:285-291.

84.   Lundberg C, Martinez-Serrano A, Cattaneo E, et al: Survival, integration, and differentiation of neural stem cell lines after transplantation to the adult rat striatum. *Exp Neurol* 1997;145(2 pt 1):342-360.

85.   Bakay RA, Raiser CD, Stover NP, et al: Implantation of Spheramine in advanced Parkinson's disease (PD). *Front Biosci* 2004; 9:592-602.

86.   Suhr ST, Gage FH: Gene therapy for neurologic disease. *Arch Neurol* 1993;50:1252-1268.

87.   Levivier M, Przedborski S, Bencsics C, et al: Intrastriatal implantation of fibroblasts genetically engineered to produce brain-derived neurotrophic factor prevents degeneration of dopaminergic neurons in a rat model of Parkinson's disease. *J Neurosci* 1995;15:7810-7820.

88.   Lundberg C, Horellou P, Mallet J, et al: Generation of DOPA-producing astrocytes by retroviral transduction of the human tyrosine hydroxylase gene: in vitro characterization and in vivo effects in the rat Parkinson model. *Exp Neurol* 1996;139:39-53.

89.   Kang UJ: Potential of gene therapy for Parkinson's disease: neurobiologic issues and new developments in gene transfer methodologies. *Mov Disord* 1998;13(suppl 1):59-72.

90.   Cao L, Zheng ZC, Zhao YC, et al: Gene therapy of Parkinson disease model rat by direct injection of plasmid DNA-lipofectin complex. *Hum Gene Ther* 1995;6:1497-1501.

91.   Choi-Lundberg DL, Lin Q, Chang YN, et al: Dopaminergic neurons protected from degeneration by GDNF gene therapy. *Science* 1997;275:838-841.

92.   Fink DJ, DeLuca NA, Goins WF, et al: Gene transfer to neurons using herpes simplex virus-based vectors. *Annu Rev Neurosci* 1996;19:265-287.

93.   Mandel RJ, Rendahl KG, Snyder RO, et al: Progress in direct striatal delivery of L-dopa via gene therapy for treatment of Parkinson's disease using recombinant adeno-associated viral vectors. *Exp Neurol* 1999;159:47-64.

94.   Fiegin A, Kaplitt M, During M, et al: Gene therapy for Parkinson's disease with AAV-GAD: An open-label, dose escalation, safety-tolerability trial. *Mov Disord* 2005;20:1236.

95.   Gash DM, Zhang Z, Ovadia A, et al: Functional recovery in parkinsonian monkeys treated with GDNF. *Nature* 1996;380:252-255.

96.   Grondin R, Gash DM: Glial cell line-derived neurotrophic factor (GDNF): a drug candidate for the treatment of Parkinson's disease. *J Neurol* 1998;245(11 suppl 3):P35-P42.

97.   Kordower JH, Palfi S, Chen E-Y, et al: Clinicopathological findings following intraventricular glial-derived neurotrophic factor treatment in a patient with Parkinson's disease. *Ann Neurol* 1999;46:419-424.

98.   Lang AE, Gill S, Patel NK, et al: Randomized controlled trial of intraputamenal glial cell line-derived neurotrophic factor infusion in Parkinson disease. *Ann Neurol* 2006;59:459-466.

99.   Freeman TB, Vawter DE, Leaverton PE, et al: Use of placebo surgery in controlled trials of a cellular-based therapy for Parkinson's disease. *N Engl J Med* 1999;341:988-992.

Chapter 8

Nonmotor Aspects of Parkinson's Disease and Their Medical Management

C hanges in personality and psychiatric function in Parkinson's disease (PD) were recognized early in our understanding of the disease. Charcot commented on the importance of the patient's emotional state in the disease, and Parkinson himself commented on the depressed mood in PD, calling the subjects of his writing 'unhappy sufferers.'[1] Cognitive impairment, unrecognized by Parkinson, has assumed increased importance because patient survival has lengthened with effective control of motor symptoms.

The autonomic nervous system is affected in PD, producing a host of complaints from disordered gastric motility to abnormal blood-pressure regulation, bladder, and sexual function. Most patients complain of vague and poorly localized symptoms (ie, fatigue, pain), which can produce significant disability. A cross-sectional study in 99 subjects with PD assessed the frequency of five nonmotor symptoms: anxiety, depression, fatigue, sleep disturbance, and sensory symptoms. All but 12% had at least one of these symptoms, 59% had two or more, and 25% had five or more.[2]

Dopaminergic treatment is unlikely to improve most of the nonmotor symptoms of PD. Moreover, the treatment of PD may exacerbate autonomic or other symptoms and may produce a spectrum of psychiatric disorders ranging from sleep disorders to frank psychosis. These important aspects of PD are significant contributors to overall disability in PD but are often given inadequate attention in both the medical literature and in the physician's office.

Personality Changes

A characteristic premorbid personality has been described in PD. Patients are with PD typically introverted, punctual, accurate, and inflexible. They have reduced initiative and motivation, and suffer from social withdrawal, fatigue, dependence, indecisiveness, and apprehension. They eschew risky behaviors and are usually involved in stable work and family situations.[3,4] These traits antedate disease onset by decades and become more prominent as the disease progresses. One positive aspect of this personality structure is that PD patients often are compliant with medication and other therapies. They also often have competent and devoted caregivers.

Depression

Depression affects 40% to 70% of PD patients. Mood disorders range from mild dysthymic disorder to major affective disorder. Only about 50% of PD patients meet the full criteria for major depression.[5] Suicidal ideation is more common than a suicide attempt or a successful suicide. The prevalence of depression has a bimodal distribution, peaking in early-onset mild disease and then again in advanced severe disease. Depression may precede motor involvement in PD, reflecting early degenerative changes in the lower brainstem regions.[6] Women and patients with early-onset PD are especially prone to depression. Other identified risk factors include right-sided symptom predominance, prominent akinesia, severe disability, and comorbid anxiety or psychosis. Depression may be difficult to diagnose in PD because many patients do not complain about depressed mood, and other symptoms often resemble psychomotor retardation.[7] A recent evidence-based review found that the

Beck Depression Inventory, Hamilton Dementia Rating Scale, and Montgomery-Asberg Depression Rating Scale may be useful screening tools in this population.[8]

For mild depression associated with adjustment to diagnosis or disability, psychological counseling and support groups can be helpful. When control of motor symptoms is suboptimal, the institution or optimization of dopaminergic therapy may also improve mood. Selegiline (Eldepryl®, Zelapar®) has some mild antidepressant properties, as well as some mild antiparkinsonian properties. At this time, the evidence does support the use of amitriptyline for depression in PD.[8] However, selective serotonin reuptake inhibitors (SSRIs) have largely overtaken tricyclic antidepressants (TCAs) for the treatment of depression in general, and they are widely used in clinical practice in depressed patients with PD.[5] In a few cases, there have been reports of serotonin syndrome in patients treated with TCAs or SSRIs concurrently with selegiline, and the product labeling cautions against the concurrent use of selegiline and SSRIs. Although a survey of movement disorders specialists suggested that serotonin syndrome occurred rarely, physicians prescribing these drugs in combination should proceed with caution.[9,10] The product labeling for rasagiline (Azilect®) specifically warns against using this agent in combination with SSRIs.[11] At least 14 days should elapse between discontinuation of rasagiline and initiation of treatment with a TCA, a SSRI, or a serotonin/norepinephrine reuptake inhibitor (SNRI) antidepressant. Because of the long half-lives of fluoxetine (Prozac®, Prozac® Weekly™, Sarafem®) and its active metabolite, at least 5 weeks (perhaps longer, especially if fluoxetine has been prescribed chronically and/or at higher doses) should elapse between discontinuation of fluoxetine and initiation of rasagiline.[11] Nonselective monoamine oxidase (MAO) inhibitors may be useful for refractory depression in patients who are not taking levodopa but are contraindicated in levodopa-treated patients because of the risk of hypertensive crisis.[7] In severely depressed patients, electroconvulsive therapy has proven useful. Anecdotal literature suggests that electroconvulsive therapy also improves motor function.[9] Experimental studies have suggested that transcranial magnetic stimulation might improve depressive symptoms in patients with PD, but this technique is not clinically available.[9]

Fatigue

Fatigue is a common complaint among PD patients, reported in 33% to 58% of patients. Patients complain of tiredness, low energy, or exhaustion. These experiences are universally related as severe and unpleasant, and they adversely affect quality of life and the activities of daily life. Symptoms of fatigue frequently overlap with depression, sleepiness, poor nocturnal sleep, apathy, and anxiety, but fatigue does seem to be an independent feature of the illness.[12] It is clear that fatigue is an important symptom of PD, and that more research is required if we are to understand its genesis and the optimal approach to its treatment.

Cognitive Impairment and Dementia

Generalized dementia is rare in early PD, and its presence in a mildly disabled patient always suggests an alternative or comorbid diagnosis. However, impairments in cognitive functions are common in PD. Interestingly, there is some evidence that cognitive impairment relates to the phenotypic expression of PD. Patients with tremor as the predominant symptom tend to have less cognitive impairment than patients with prominent bradykinesia and rigidity.[13] Cognitive impairment also appears prominent in patients whose symptoms began on the left side.[14] Even early in PD, most patients complain that there have been changes in cognitive function. Most patients also complain that they have difficulty with organizing, planning, and multitasking. Measures of executive function—including anticipation, goal selection, planning, monitoring, and use of feedback—have consistently shown deficits, even in early PD. Additionally, decision-making time appears to be longer in PD than in normal control subjects.[13] These deficits do not respond to dopaminergic therapy. Patients and their families are understandably concerned about cognitive dysfunction and must be assured that these problems are common and do not necessarily portend the development of frank dementia. Patients and family members also should be urged to use strategies to focus attention, such as turning off the television or putting down the newspaper during conversations, writing reminders, and developing easily remembered routines.

Prevalence estimates for dementia in PD vary from 28% to 78%, increasing with disease duration.[15] Risk factors for the development of dementia in PD include older age, family history of dementia, greater motor impairment, lower education status, and psychiatric complications of dopaminergic therapy. The classification of PD dementia is evolving. A subgroup of patients have comorbid Alzheimer's disease (AD), and show typical cognitive changes including prominent memory loss and disorders of language and praxis. However, for most demented parkinsonian patients, the underlying pathology shows Lewy body involvement of the cerebral cortex. Clinically, dementia associated with diffuse Lewy body disease (DLBD) is usually characterized by disorders of attention, concentration, mood, and retrieval of learned material. Within the context of Lewy body dementia, the differentiation between dementia associated with PD and DLBD is an evolving concept. DLBD is generally diagnosed when dementia and parkinsonism begin within 1 year of each other, and the patient shows other characteristic features, such as early hallucinations, even in the absence of dopaminergic therapy, exquisite sensitivity to neuroleptics, and spontaneous fluctuations in alertness and cognition.[16] Patients in whom a long motor course typical of PD is complicated by the late development of cognitive impairment with confusion and hallucinations are usually considered to have dementia associated with PD. The reader should note that the evolution of this concept continues.[17] Whatever the root cause, dementia in PD does not improve with dopaminergic pharmacotherapy, and it is a risk factor for central dopaminergic complications, such as psychosis, and ultimately, for nursing home placement and death.

Because PD patients have cholinergic deficits, cholinesterase inhibitors have been studied for cognitive impairment in PD. The evidence base supports the efficacy of both donepezil (Aricept®) and rivastigmine (Exelon®, Exelon® Patch) for the treatment of cognitive impairment in PD. The effects of cholinesterase inhibiton in PD is modest, and patients must be watched for signs of increased tremor during therapy.[18]

Sleep Disruption

Between 60% and 98% of outpatients with PD report one or more sleep abnormalities, and almost 50% take sleep medications. Sleep disorders relate to the underlying pathophysiology of PD and to pathologic involvement of the brainstem but also relate to medications and other medical illnesses. In some patients, sleep complaints precede the onset of PD. Excessive daytime sleepiness is common in PD and may relate to poor nocturnal sleep or to the effects of the underlying PD or of medications. PD patients have less total sleep time, slow-wave sleep, non-rapid eye movement (NREM) sleep, and sleep efficiency.[19] A common complaint is fragmented sleep. PD patients generally do not have difficulty falling asleep, but, after an initial sleep period of one to several hours, reawaken every 1 to 2 hours.[20] Reasons given for these awakenings vary. Some patients report that they awaken because immobility impairs the ability to turn in bed or adjust the bedclothes (ie, nocturnal akinesia). Others have dystonic leg cramps related to dopaminergic therapy withdrawal. Many complain of nocturia.[21] Another frequent nocturnal complaint is altered dreaming, reported by about 50% of patients. These altered dreams are vivid, brightly colored, and may be more involved and bizarre than earlier-life dreams.[20] PD patients also have a higher prevalence of rapid eye movement (REM) behavior disorder (RBD). RBD sufferers do not have the normal skeletal muscle paralysis associated with REM sleep and, thus, may thrash, kick, hit, or otherwise 'act out' their dreams. Typical RBD symptoms may precede the development of PD or other parkinsonisms or may occur during the course of the illness.[22] In a recent survey, 15% of PD patients had behaviors typically seen in RBD, and in 33% of patients, sleep-related behaviors had resulted in an injury to themselves or their bed partners.[23] Sleep hygiene, comorbid medical disorders, and the effects of medication must also be considered.

Restless legs syndrome (RLS), which is known to be related to dopaminergic mechanisms in the general population, may occur with increased frequency in patients with PD. Typically, patients with RLS complain of uncomfortable sensations of restlessness in their legs that are relieved only by moving their legs about. It is important to recognize sleep disorders that have a significant negative impact on quality of life in PD.[21]

Treatment of sleep disorders in PD can be difficult. Good sleep hygiene and regular bedtime routines should be encouraged. Alcohol (ethanol) should be avoided late in the day because it tends to increase sleep fragmentation. Patients with clear symptoms related to immobility, dystonia, or restless legs usually benefit from an increase in dopaminergic therapy, such as the addition of controlled-release carbidopa/levodopa (Sinemet® CR) at bedtime. Sleep fragmentation often responds to an additional small dose of antidepressant, such as amitriptyline or trazodone, at bedtime. Nocturia may respond to oral medications, such as oxybutynin (Ditropan®, Ditropan XL®) or tolterodine (Detrol®, Detrol® LA), or to intranasal desmopressin (Stimate®).[21] Altered dreams should signal the treating physician to

Table 8-1: Sleep Disorders and Their Treatment

Disorder	Drug	Dose Range
Nocturnal akinesia	Controlled-release carbidopa/levodopa (Sinemet® CR)	25/100-50/200 mg at bedtime
Sleep fragmentation	Amitriptyline	10-50 mg at bedtime
	Trazodone	50-100 mg at bedtime
Vivid dreams (if severe)	Quetiapine* (Seroquel®)	12.5-25 mg at bedtime
Rapid eye movement (REM) behavior disorder (RBD)	Clonazepam (Klonopin®)	0.25-1 mg at bedtime

*Not FDA approved for use in sleep disorders

exercise caution in increasing the dose of dopaminergic medications and to be alert for the development of hallucinations. A small dose of an atypical antipsychotic, such as quetiapine (Seroquel®), may be useful in distressing cases. RBD responds to low doses of clonazepam (Klonopin®) taken at bedtime (Table 8-1).

Drug-induced Hallucinations and Psychosis

Psychotic symptoms were rarely mentioned in PD before the 1960s, suggesting that those symptoms relate to dopaminergic treatment. Hallucinations and delusions are serious signs in PD because their presence best predicts the need for institutionalization and, once institutionalized, mortality among these patients is extremely high.[24,25] Hallucinations are seen in 8% to 40% of PD patients on chronic dopaminergic therapy.[26] In PD, hallucinations usually begin after 1 year, and commonly after 3 to 5 years of levodopa therapy. The development of hallucinations within the first year of levodopa monotherapy is atypical and raises the possibility of an alternate diagnosis, particularly DLBD, concomitant primary psychiatric disease, or AD.[27] Dopamine agonist monotherapy is associated with a higher risk of hallucinations in the first year (ie, as many as 10% of patients), and it is not yet known whether this suggests an alternate diagnosis.[28,29]

The hallucinations of chronically treated PD are rather stereotyped. They are usually visual, nonthreatening, and brightly colored. People and animals figure prominently. These hallucinations are often familiar to the patient and may be friends, workmates, and family members. There is a distinct illusory quality to the hallucinations—an existing stimulus, such as a floor lamp or humped up bedclothes, may take on an animate appearance. The faces are often obscured, and although the patient may try to interact with them, the hallucinations do not speak or make noise. These hallucinations are particularly common in the evening and at night and often recur in the same areas in the house. They also occur in the context of a clear sensorium. Nonvisual hallucinations are somewhat less common, and may occur in the context of an acute confusional state, such as during acute illness or hospitalization. Alternatively, they may suggest more widespread neuropathology, such as DLBD, concomitant AD, or primary psychopathology.[27]

Once hallucinations appear, they tend to persist absent any intervention.[20] Chronic hallucinations may become more threatening, and the patient may lose insight that the visions are not real and may take action against the hallucinations. As many as 10% of chronically treated PD patients also will develop drug-induced delusions, typically that a spouse is unfaithful or family or friends are stealing money or possessions. In this stage in the evolution of drug-induced psychosis, the patient may telephone the police or take other action based upon their hallucinations or delusions. At this point, urgent intervention may be required.

Assessment and Management of Drug-induced Psychotic Symptoms

Many patients do not spontaneously discuss benign hallucinations at a routine office visit, so the treating physician must ask about them at each office visit. Because hallucinations are more common in patients with cognitive impairment, cognitive functions should be assessed in patients who begin to hallucinate. Benign hallucinations with retained insight can be followed conservatively. The patient and family members should be instructed to contact the physician if the hallucinations become threatening, insight is lost, or delusions appear. Figure 8-1 outlines the stepwise treatment for more serious hallucinations. First, extraneous medications, including hypnosedatives, anxiolytics, anticholinergics, amantadine, and catechol-o-methyl transferase (COMT) inhibitors should be discontinued. Next, direct-acting dopamine agonists should be reduced or eliminated. Levodopa can be reduced to the lowest level that allows functional independence. If hallucinations or delusions persist following these changes, an antipsychotic should be added. Typical antipsychotics, such as haloperidol (Haldol®) and thioridazine, worsen mobility and are not indicated in these patients. The newer atypical antipsychotics, particularly quetiapine and clozapine (Clozaril®), have been shown in anecdotal reports to improve hallucinations without significantly worsening parkinsonian symptoms.[30,31] However, the accumulating evidence base supports only clozapine for the treatment of drug-induced psychosis in PD.[32] About 85% of psychotic PD patients can successfully be controlled with clozapine, without worsening of motor function. The effective dose range is 12.5 to 50 mg/day given as

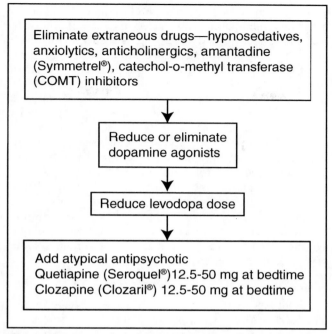

Figure 8-1: Treatment of drug-induced psychotic symptoms.

a nighttime dose. The average effective dose is 25 mg.[33] However, because clozapine is associated with hematopoietic toxicity, and requires frequent monitoring of the patient's blood count, most clinicians prefer to use other atypical drugs. Of the other available agents, quetiapine most closely resembles clozapine. Quetiapine appears somewhat less efficacious than clozapine for controlling psychosis and has a greater propensity to worsen motor function. However, because it is easier to use than clozapine, most clinicians consider quetiapine the drug of choice for treating psychosis in PD. The effective dose range is generally between 12.5 and 67.5 mg/day given as a nighttime dose. Patients who fail quetiapine should be given a therapeutic trial of clozapine, beginning with 6.25 mg at bedtime and increasing as needed to the range of 25 to 75 mg at bedtime. Risperidone (Risperdal®) and olanzapine (Zyprexa®) have been poorly tolerated in small studies in PD and are generally not recommended for the treatment of psychosis in PD. Ziprasidone (Geodon®) has not been studied in PD.[33] The serotonin 5-HT3 antagonist ondansetron (Zofran®, Zofran ODT®) has been studied in a small study and was found to improve psychosis in PD, but the results have not been confirmed and the agent is far too expensive for routine use. The cholinesterase inhibitors galantamine (Razadyne®, Razadyne® ER), rivastigmine and donepezil have had limited study for the treatment of psychosis in PD but may be useful in some patients.[33] Generally, treatment of drug-induced psychotic symptoms can be carried out at home, although some psychotic patients may require hospitalization.

Fatigue

About 50% of PD patients report feeling fatigued, compared with <20% of controls.[34] Fatigue is the most troublesome symptom in 33% of patients.[35] Compared with patients without fatigue, PD patients with fatigue have depression, cognitive impairment, longer duration and more severe disease, higher levodopa dose, and greater use of hypnosedatives. Although depression correlates best with fatigue in PD, many nondepressed patients also endorse this symptom. Motor control testing confirms a 50% increase in fatigue in performance of a continuous motor task in subjects with PD compared with age-matched controls. Fatigue in this study improved with levodopa administration, suggesting this symptom is related to the underlying dopamine deficiency state.[36] Considered together, these findings suggest that the appropriate use of antidopaminergic therapy, identification and treatment of depression, and optimization of sleep patterns can best manage fatigue.

Pain

Pain is a symptom of PD that is frequently overlooked. A survey of 123 patients with PD reported a median number of two pains per patient. Eighty-five percent of patients reported a problem with pain, and nearly 30% had four or more pains. Pain was directly related to PD in almost 63% of patients and indirectly related to PD in about 10%.[37] PD-related pain is often severe during maximal motor disability. Pain can be clinically classified as musculoskeletal, neuritic, or radicular, associated with dystonia, primary or central pain, or pain associated with motor restlessness (ie, akathisia).[38] Depression may contribute to pain, but is rarely the sole cause of the complaint. The treatment of pain in PD involves identifying and treating any underlying source of tissue injury, such as spinal stenosis, deformity, or arthritis. Antiparkinsonian therapies should be optimized, and antidepressants initiated, if indicated. Symptomatic treatments for pain, such as nonsteroidal anti-inflammatory drugs (NSAIDs), may be used if appropriate.

Autonomic Dysfunction

Autonomic dysfunction is an important clinical sign in PD. When it occurs early and is a prominent feature of a parkinsonian illness, it should lead the clinician to consider alternative diagnoses, particularly the autonomic subtype of multiple-system atrophy. With the advancement of PD, however, autonomic symptoms often emerge, although they rarely reach a magnitude similar to that seen in multiple-system atrophy. Frequent autonomic complaints relate to bladder and sexual dysfunction, orthostatic hypotension, slowed gastrointestinal (GI) transport, and excessive perspiration. Seventy percent to 90% of PD patients have one or more autonomic complaints.[39,40] Neuropathologic studies confirm the presence of neurodegeneration with Lewy body formation in the hypothalamus, and sympathetic and parasympathetic autonomic ganglia in PD accounting for the frequency of GI complaints.[41]

Common complaints related to drooling, dysphagia, postprandial bloating, and constipation occur in about 75% of patients. Urinary complaints, especially urgency, increased frequency of micturition, or incontinence related to detrusor hyperreflexia are experienced by 35% to 70% of patients. About 60% of men complain of impotence, whereas 15% of all PD patients have symptoms referable to cardiovascular instability, such as orthostatic hypotension.[42] Other complaints include paroxysmal or constant excessive perspiration over the head and torso, and disordered thermoregulation.

Antiparkinsonian drugs can worsen autonomic complaints. Anticholinergic drugs typically worsen constipation and other signs of impaired GI motility. Levodopa and direct-acting dopamine agonists can induce or worsen GI complaints or orthostatic hypotension, as can concomitant medications, such as antidepressants or hypnosedatives.

Treatment of Autonomic Complaints

Although not an approved indication by the US Food and Drug Administration (FDA), drooling can be treated with peripherally acting anticholinergic drugs, such as glycopyrrolate (Robinul®, Robinul® Forte) or propantheline (Pro-Banthine®). Botulinum toxin, especially serotype B (Myobloc®), injections into the salivary glands have recently been suggested to lessen drooling in refractory cases, but this is not a FDA-approved usage of the drug.[43] Dysphagia should be assessed by a speech therapist, and it often will require a bedside or radiologic swallowing assessment. Speech therapists can often suggest swallowing strategies that improve swallowing efficiency and safety or can prescribe helpful dietary changes. Some patients will require artificial feeding. Although metoclopramide (Reglan®) is often used to improve symptoms of poor upper GI motility in the nonparkinsonian population, this agent worsens parkinsonism and must be avoided. Bloating and delayed gastric emptying can be controlled with domperidone, a peripheral dopamine antagonist shown to be safe in PD. However, domperidone is not available in the United States. Constipation responds partially to increases in dietary fiber, water consumption, and exercise. A daily stool softener as well as herbal remedies, such as senna-containing teas or other concoctions, may also be useful. A fruit paste containing senna (Table 8-2) can be prepared at home and is well tolerated and effective in PD. Cathartic agents should be avoided whenever possible but often become necessary in longstanding cases of constipation. Oxybutynin and tolterodine are also useful for symptoms of overactive bladder (OAB). Symptomatic orthostatic hypotension should prompt a thorough evaluation of all medications. Because peripheral conversion of levodopa to dopamine can worsen hypotension, the carbidopa dose should be increased to at least 100 mg daily. Dopamine agonist therapy should be re-examined. Patients should be told to dangle their legs over the side of the bed before arising and to change positions gradually. Conservative measures for hypotension include adding sodium and caffeine to the diet, sleeping with the head of the bed elevated 30%, and wearing elastic stockings. Residual hypotension can be treated with fludrocortisone. When hypotension is severe, sympathomimetic agents, such as midodrine (Pro-Amatine®), may be required.

Vision Complaints

Patients with PD frequently complain about poor visual function, including blurred vision, difficulty reading, and less commonly, diplopia. Deficits in visual function are poorly understood by most clinicians, and these complaints are frequently ignored or attributed to antiparkinsonian medications. A visual assessment by an optometrist or ophthalmologist often has shown no significant reduction in visual acuity. Other deficiencies in visual function have been well documented in the clinical literature. The basal ganglia are important in the control of extraocular

Table 8-2: Anticonstipation Fruit Paste

1 lb pitted prunes

1 lb raisins

1 lb figs

1 3.5 to 4 oz package of senna tea (from health food store)

1 cup brown sugar

1 cup lemon juice

Prepare tea: use 3.5 cups boiling water to a package of tea; steep 5 minutes.

Strain tea and add 2 cups to large pot. Add fruit. Boil tea and fruit for 5 minutes. Remove from heat. Add sugar and lemon juice. Cool. Puree in food processor or blender.

Take 1 to 2 tbs daily. Can be frozen in glass jars or plastic containers.

movements, and patients with PD may have difficulties generating voluntary REM. Contrast sensitivity and color vision are impaired in PD, and the ability to detect motion may also be impaired.[44] Reading in PD is difficult because these patients have trouble generating repetitive REM and refixations, and have difficulty suppressing visual information from the last eye position. Additionally, difficulty with convergent eye movement causes blurring or frank diplopia during reading. Although many of these deficits relate to dopamine deficiency in the striatum or the retina, visual complaints are only partially responsive to antiparkinsonian medications. Visual cues, such as following text with a finger, may facilitate saccades and refixation. Bifocal lenses are difficult to use for patients with oculomotor deficits and should be abandoned in favor of separate pairs of glasses with single-vision lenses for nearsighted and farsighted vision. Task lighting should be bright to facilitate contrast. Exercises to strengthen convergent eye movements may be helpful. 'Pencil push-ups' are such an exercise. The patient focuses on the tip of a pencil held at arm's length and slowly brings the pencil toward the nose, maintaining its tip in focus. Depending on the degree and constancy of diplopia, some patients can be treated with prisms. This usually requires the attention of a neuro-ophthalmologist. When all else fails, the patient can patch one eye to improve reading.

References

1. Parkinson J: *An Essay on the Shaking Palsy.* London, England, Whittingham and Rowland, 1817.

2. Shulman LM, Taback RL, Bean J, et al: Comorbidity of the nonmotor symptoms of Parkinson's disease. *Mov Disord* 2001;16: 507-510.

3. Todes CJ, Lees AJ: The pre-morbid personality of patients with Parkinson's disease. *J Neurol Neurosurg Psychiatry* 1985;48: 97-100.

4. Cote L: Depression: impact and management by the patient and family. *Neurology* 1999;52(7 suppl 3):S7-S9.

5. Sawabini KA, Watts RL: Treatment of depression in Parkinson's disease. *Parkinsonism Related Disord* 2004;10(suppl 1):S37-S41.

6. Braak H, Del Tredici K, Rub U, et al: Staging of brain pathology related to sporadic Parkinson's disease. *Neurobiol Aging* 2003; 24:197-211.

7. Poewe W, Luginger E: Depression in Parkinson's disease: impediments to recognition and treatment options. *Neurology* 1999; 52(7 suppl 3):S2-S6.

8. Miyasaki JM, Shannon K, Voon V, Quality Standards Subcommittee of the American Academy of Neurology, et al: Practice Parameter: evaluation and treatment of depression, psychosis, and dementia in Parkinson's disease (an evidence-based review): report of the quality standards subcommittee of the American Academy of Neurology. *Neurology* 2006;66:996-1002.

9.   Tom T, Cummings JL: Depression in Parkinson's disease. Pharmacological characteristics and treatment. *Drugs Aging* 1998;12: 55-74.

10.   Heinonen EH, Myllyla V: Safety of selegiline (deprenyl) in the treatment of Parkinson's disease. *Drug Saf* 1998;19:11-22.

11.   Azilect® Package Insert. Teva Pharmaceutical Industries Ltd, Kfar Saba, Israel, 2006.

12.   Friedman JH, Brown RG, Comella C, et al: Fatigue in Parkinson's disease: A review. *Mov Disord* 2007;22:297-308.

13.   Levin BE, Katzen HL: Early cognitive changes and nondementing behavioral abnormalities in Parkinson's disease. *Adv Neurol* 2005;96:84-94.

14.   Tomer R, Levin BE, Weiner WJ: Side of onset of motor symptoms influences cognition in Parkinson's disease. *Ann Neurol* 1993;34:579-584.

15.   Aarsland D, Zaccai J, Brayne C: A systematic review of prevalence studies of dementia in Parkinson's disease. *Mov Disord* 2005;20:1255-1263.

16.   McKeith IG, Dickson DW, Lowe J, Consortium on DLB, et al: Diagnosis and management of dementia with Lewy bodies: third report of the DLB consortium. *Neurology* 2005;65:1863-1872.

17.   Lippa CF, Duda JE, Grossman M, et al, and the DLB/PDD Working Group: DLB and PDD boundary issues: diagnosis, treatment, molecular pathology, and biomarkers. *Neurology* 2007;68:812-819.

18.   Leroi I, Collins D, Marsh L, et al: Non-dopaminergic treatment of cognitive impairment and dementia in Parkinson's disease: a review. *J Neurol Sci* 2006;248:104-114.

19.   Adler CH, Thorpy MJ: Sleep issues in Parkinson's disease. *Neurology* 2005;64(12 suppl 3):S12-S20.

20.   Pappert EJ, Goetz CG, Niederman FG, et al: Hallucinations, sleep fragmentation, and altered dream phenomena in Parkinson's disease. *Mov Disord* 1999;14:117-121.

21.   Partinen M: Sleep disorder related to Parkinson's disease. *J Neurol* 1997;244(4 suppl 1):S3-S6.

22.   Schenck CH, Bundlie SR, Mahowald MW: Delayed emergence of a parkinsonian disorder in 38% of 29 older men initially diagnosed with idiopathic rapid eye movement sleep behaviour disorder. *Neurology* 1996;46:388-393.

23. Comella CL, Nardine TM, Diederich NJ, et al: Sleep-related violence, injury, and REM sleep behavior disorder in Parkinson's disease. *Neurology* 1998;51:526-529.

24. Goetz CG, Stebbins GT: Risk factors for nursing home placement in advanced Parkinson's disease. *Neurology* 1993;43:2227-2229.

25. Goetz CG, Stebbins GT: Mortality and hallucinations in nursing home patients with advanced Parkinson's disease. *Neurology* 1995;45:669-671.

26. Barnes J, David AS: Visual hallucinations in Parkinson's disease: a review and phenomenological survey. *J Neurol Neurosurg Psychiatry* 2001;70:727-733.

27. Goetz CG, Vogel C, Tanner CM, et al: Early dopaminergic drug-induced hallucinations in parkinsonian patients. *Neurology* 1998;51:811-814.

28. Shannon KM, Bennett JP Jr, Friedman JH: Efficacy of pramipexole, a novel dopamine agonist, as monotherapy in mild to moderate Parkinson's disease. The Pramipexole Study Group. *Neurology* 1997;49:724-728.

29. Adler CH, Sethi KD, Hauser RA, et al: Ropinirole for the treatment of early Parkinson's disease. The Ropinirole Study Group. *Neurology* 1997;49:393-399.

30. Aarsland D, Larsen JP, Lim NG, et al: Olanzapine for psychosis in patients with Parkinson's disease with and without dementia. *J Neuropsychiatry Clin Neurosci* 1999;11:392-394.

31. Fernandez HH, Friedman JH, Jacques C, et al: Quetiapine for the treatment of drug-induced psychosis in Parkinson's disease. *Mov Disord* 1999;14:484-487.

32. Frieling H, Hillemacher T, Ziegenbein M, et al: Treating dopamimetic psychosis in Parkinson's disease: structured review and meta-analysis. *Eur Neuropsychopharmacol* 2007;17:165-171.

33. Wint DP, Okun MS, Fernandez HH: Psychosis in Parkinson's Disease. *J Geriatr Psychiatry Neurol* 2004;17:127-136.

34. Karlsen K, Larsen JP, Tandberg E, et al: Fatigue in patients with Parkinson's disease. *Mov Disord* 1999;14:237-241.

35. Friedman J, Friedman H: Fatigue in Parkinson's disease. *Neurology* 1993;43:2016-2018.

36.   Ziv I, Avraham M, Michaelov Y, et al: Enhanced fatigue during motor performance in patients with Parkinson's disease. *Neurology* 1998;51:1583-1586.

37.   Lee MA, Walker RW, Hildreth TJ, et al: A survey of pain in idiopathic Parkinson's disease. *J Pain Symptom Manage* 2006:32: 462-469.

38.   Ford B: Pain in Parkinson's disease. *Clin Neurosci* 1998;5:63-72.

39.   Magalhaes M, Wenning GK, Daniel SE, et al: Autonomic dysfunction in pathologically confirmed multiple system atrophy and idiopathic Parkinson's disease—a retrospective comparison. *Acta Neurol Scand* 1995;91:98-102.

40.   Singer C, Weiner WJ, Sanchez-Ramos JR: Autonomic dysfunction in men with Parkinson's disease. *Eur Neurol* 1992;32:134-140.

41.   Wakabayashi K, Takahashi H: Neuropathology of autonomic nervous system in Parkinson's disease. *Eur Neurol* 1997;38(suppl 2): 2-7.

42.   Martignoni E, Pacchetti C, Godi L, et al: Autonomic disorders in Parkinson's disease. *J Neural Transm Suppl* 1995;45:11-19.

43.   Pal PK, Calne DB, Calne S, et al: Botulinum toxin A as treatment for drooling saliva in PD. *Neurology* 2000;54:244-247.

44.   Hunt LA, Sadun AA, Bassi CJ: Review of the visual system in Parkinson's disease. *Optom Vis Sci* 1995;72:92-99.

Chapter 9

Other Treatment Modalities

Frustration with the limitations of medical and surgical therapy to treat Parkinson's disease (PD) fuels the search for new treatment strategies. Ancillary medical therapies—including physical, occupational, and speech therapy—play increasingly important roles for patients as the disease advances. Chiropractic manipulation frequently relieves rigidity or musculoskeletal complaints, and, in rare cases, reports suggest that it improves signs and symptoms of PD. Herbal and natural remedies are attractive to patients, although few of these remedies have been subjected to rigorous studies that include the use of comparison groups. As a result, the role of natural remedies remains poorly defined, and little information is available to guide the physician in incorporating them into daily practice.

Ancillary Therapies

Physical therapy

Physical therapy is commonly prescribed in PD, particularly when treatment-resistant gait disability, freezing, and postural instability threaten a patient's safety. A review of the evidence regarding the efficacy of physical therapy concluded that most studies showed improvement in outcomes with this intervention.[1] The focus of physical therapy changes across the course of the disease. Early in PD, physical therapy focuses on increasing strength and stability, maximizing the efficiency of gait, and optimizing posture and balance. In moderate-to-advanced disease, improving range of motion and preventing falls and other complications of decreased mobility are a valuable supplement to medical therapy. During this time, many patients require assessments for and training in the appropriate use of walking aids, such as canes and walkers. In late disease, therapy focuses on maintaining range of motion and reducing the complications of immobility.[2]

It is usually not possible to obtain third-party payment for continuous physical therapy in patients with chronic progressive illnesses, but PD patients often benefit from intermittent physical therapy and continuous home exercise programs. Walking is particularly helpful, and most patients are able to maintain a walking program involving a daily 1-mile walk or more. Weight training exercises are often recommended to improve posture and maintain functional skills, but the benefit of these exercises remains unproven. Patients should be supervised when engaged in weight training to ensure that exercises are performed properly.

In-patient physical rehabilitation is valuable for PD patients recovering from a hip fracture or other illness because these patients recover more slowly than nonparkinsonian patients of similar age.[3]

Occupational therapy

Occupational therapy is a valuable supplement to physical therapy, particularly when activities of daily living become impaired. A randomized, controlled trial of group occupational therapy in PD demonstrated improvements in bradykinesia and psychological well-being in the treated group that persisted for 12 months after completion of therapy.[4] Because occupational therapy is often prescribed in conjunction with physical and speech therapy, it may be difficult to clinically separate its benefits. Periodic driving skills assessments, offered at many comprehensive rehabilitation centers, are helpful in advising patients about their ability to safely operate a motor vehicle.

Speech therapy

Speech and swallowing complaints are common in PD. Seventy percent of patients complain of disordered speech or swallowing, and 29% identify these complaints as among their most disturbing symptoms.[5] Speech in PD is characterized by reduced loudness, reduced pitch inflection, reduced range of articulatory motions, short rushes of speech, and stuttering.[5] Typical signs of swallowing dysfunction in PD include drooling, pills getting stuck in the throat, labored eating, choking or coughing after swallowing, weight loss, and aspiration pneumonia. A cross-sectional study showed dysphagia in 30% of unselected patients attending a university clinic, and the study found no clinical predictors for its presence.[6] These midline signs of PD often poorly respond to dopaminergic therapy.[7] Both may improve with speech therapy.

Speech therapy addresses two major areas of speech disability in PD: impaired phonation and impaired articulation. A number of open-label trials showed improvements in speech intelligibility following various speech therapy interventions, but speech therapy has been considered to have poor carryover into everyday speech and poor long-term benefits. Two specific speech therapy techniques, the Lee Silverman Voice Treatment (LSVT), which focuses on high-effort loud phonation to improve respiration, phonation, and articulation, and the Pitch Limiting Voice Treatment (PLVT), which focuses on speaking loudly, but with a lower pitch, have been shown to improve loudness in PD.[8]

Swallowing dysfunction is common in PD. Patients should be routinely queried about difficulty swallowing food because no other clinical criterion predicts who is at risk for dysphagia.[6] Because swallowing may partially improve with optimal dopaminergic therapy, dysphagia should prompt a careful reassessment of therapy. Optimally treated patients should receive a bedside swallowing evaluation followed by a formal radiologic swallow study. A speech therapist can often suggest strategies to improve swallowing safety and efficacy.[6] Dietary changes, including changing the consistency of solids and using thickening agents for thin liquids, may be necessary. Fortunately, progression to a need for tube feeding is uncommon.

Chiropractic manipulation

Many patients seek chiropractic manipulation to address changes in posture, gait, and balance, as well as to control the back and neck pain that are often concomitant with PD. A detailed case report suggested improvements in parkinsonian symptoms and signs in a single patient after a prolonged course of manipulation of the first cervical vertebra.[9] However, because no scientific data support the role of the cervical cord in the pathogenesis of PD, there appears to be no rationale for the efficacy of the approach. With the exception of limiting cervical manipulation in elderly patients with rheumatoid arthritis or degenerative spinal column disease, there are no contraindications to chiropractic therapy in PD.

Alternative Medicine Approaches to Parkinson's Disease

Herbal and natural remedies

Alternative health care is a booming industry in the United States. Although data specific to PD are not available, as many as 40% of US residents use alternative therapies. PD patients who use natural remedies may be embarrassed, or may feel it is not important to discuss their use of these treatments with their physicians. Patients should be encouraged to list all prescription, nonprescription, and herbal or natural remedies at each clinic visit.

Certain foods naturally contain levodopa. For example, ingestion of 250 g of broad beans significantly improves parkinsonian symptoms and increases plasma levodopa concentrations.[10] Herbal remedies most commonly used by PD patients are gingko biloba, melatonin, coenzyme Q_{10}, creatine, evening primrose, ginger, lecithin, passion flower, and St. John's wort. Some practitioners offer therapies, such as hormonal supplements and intravenous antioxidants, such as glutathione, often marketing them over the Internet. These therapies have not been shown to be effective in controlled clinical trials. It is important to realize that there is a substantial placebo effect in PD.[11] Open and anecdotal trials must be viewed with caution.

A coherent description of PD appears in the ancient medical system of Ayurveda under the name Kampavata. These traditional herbal therapies of Ayurveda contain anticholinergics, monoamine oxidase (MAO) inhibitors, and levodopa.[12] An open trial of HP-200 (derived from the traditional Ayurveda treatment *Mucuna pruriens*, which contains levodopa) of 34 levodopa-naive and 26 levodopa-treated patients suggested that HP-200 provided significant improvements in motor dysfunction.[13]

Most allopathic physicians consider alternative medicine therapies to be benign, and no published data suggest that they are detrimental to PD patients. There is insufficient foundation to recommend any particular herbal or alternative 'cocktail' to PD patients because none has been subjected to rigorous study.

Acupuncture

Acupuncture has been reported to relieve tremor, rigidity, and dyskinesia as well as improve balance and circulation in a small series of PD patients.[14] Acupuncture has not been subjected to controlled clinical trials in PD, so there is no objective foundation to recommend it as a treatment for parkinsonism.

The Physician's Approach to Ancillary Services and Alternative Therapies

Each physician must find a way to integrate nonmedical therapies into clinical practice. Ancillary therapies should be prescribed with specific goals in mind, eg, improving strength, flexibility, balance, speech and swallowing, and functional independence. A frank discussion with patients about the potential risks and benefits of poorly studied therapies will help patients to decide whether to invest in unproven alternative therapies.

References

1. Gage H, Storey L: Rehabilitation for Parkinson's disease: a systematic review of available evidence. *Clin Rehabil* 2004;18: 463-482.

2. Morris ME: Movement disorders in people with Parkinson disease: a model for physical therapy. *Phys Ther* 2000;80:578-597.

3. Jonsson B, Sernbo I, Johnell O: Rehabilitation of hip fracture patients with Parkinson's disease. *Scand J Rehabil Med* 1995;27: 227-230.

4. Gauthier L, Dalziel S, Gauthier S: The benefits of group occupational therapy for patients with Parkinson's disease. *Am J Occup Ther* 1987;41:360-365.

5. Ramig LO: How effective is the Lee Silverman voice treatment? *ASHA* 1997;39:34-35.

6. Clarke CE, Gullaksen E, Macdonald S, et al: Referral criteria for speech and language therapy assessment of dysphagia caused by idiopathic Parkinson's disease. *Acta Neurol Scand* 1998;97:27-35.

7. Kompoliti K, Wang QE, Goetz CG, et al: Effects of central dopaminergic stimulation by apomorphine on speech in Parkinson's disease. *Neurology* 2000;54:458-462.

8. de Swart BJ, Willemse SC, Maassen BA, et al: Improvement of voicing in patients with Parkinson's disease by speech therapy. *Neurology* 2003;60:498-500.

9. Elster EL: Upper cervical chiropractic management of a patient with Parkinson's disease: a case report. *J Manipulative Physiol Ther* 2000;23:573-577.

10. Rabey JM, Vered Y, Shabtai H, et al: Improvement of parkinsonian features correlate with high plasma levodopa values after broad bean (Vicia faba) consumption. *J Neurol Neurosurg Psychiatry* 1992;55:725-727.

11. Goetz CG, Leurgans S, Raman R, et al: Objective changes in motor function during placebo treatment in PD. *Neurology* 2000;54: 710-714.

12. Manyam BV, Sanchez-Ramos JR: Traditional and complementary therapies in Parkinson's disease. *Adv Neurol* 1999;80:565-574.

13. An alternative medicine treatment for Parkinson's disease: results of a multicenter clinical trial. HP-200 in Parkinson's Disease Study Group. *J Altern Complement Med* 1995;1:249-255.

14. Walton-Hadlock J: Primary Parkinson's disease: the use of Tuina and acupuncture in accord with an evolving hypothesis of its cause from the perspective of Chinese traditional medicine—Part 2. *Am J Acupunct* 1999;27:31-49.

9

Chapter 10

Summary and Other Considerations

James Parkinson's astute observations of elderly subjects in the streets of London in 1817 brought into focus the clinical syndrome characterized by mid- to late-life onset of bradykinesia, tremor, and gait disorder. More than 180 years later, we still rely on clinical criteria to diagnose Parkinson's disease (PD) and to differentiate it from other types of parkinsonism. Neuroimaging techniques now being developed may help us arrive at an objective diagnosis and improve on the sensitivity and specificity of the clinical diagnosis. We have come to understand the pathologic, physiologic, and pharmacologic bases of PD, but there is still much to learn. Recently discovered genetic abnormalities found in parkinsonism and other neurodegenerative diseases, and animal models using mitochondrial toxins, are helping us understand the importance of protein metabolism and cellular energy processes in cell degeneration. The potential ramifications of fully understanding these basic cellular processes are enormous, and are likely to lead to effective neuroprotective therapies.

Modern pharmacology continues to evolve. The introduction of levodopa to treat PD in the late 1960s allowed patients to regain a functional state, with an extended lifespan and a dramatically improved quality of life. However, this advance in treatment also revealed to us a wider spectrum of disease, because prolonging life brought with it a greater degree of degeneration before death. In addition, the nonphysiologic nature of dopamine replacement, with its short-acting precursor levodopa, changes the responsiveness of dopamine receptors themselves, and causes patients to experience motor response fluctuations, including dyskinesias, that were never a part of the underlying disease. The evolution of direct-acting dopamine agonist drugs addressed some of these problems, but no drug is as well tolerated as levodopa and none is poised to usurp its dominance in the pharmacotherapy of PD. An increased understanding of the multiple neurochemical changes in PD will undoubtedly lead to better therapies for the movement disorder. The adverse psychiatric effects of dopaminergic therapy affect a substantial minority of patients, but are important because they portend nursing home placement and death. Newer antipsychotic agents have dramatically improved the plight of hallucinating parkinsonian patients.

Surgical approaches to PD have been used for about 50 years. Before the advent of effective pharmacotherapy, surgery was the only potent treatment for parkinsonian tremor. Following the introduction of levodopa, surgery for PD became rare. The field for further surgical investigation became fertile only after chronic levodopa therapy failed and the pathophysiology of bradykinesia became more apparent.

Stimulation of deep-brain nuclei result in moderate to marked improvements of various symptoms, depending on the deep-brain target and the skill and experience of the operating team. Surgical procedures that aim to replace dopamine neurons, such as human fetal substantia nigra transplantation, have shown mixed results, achieving only modest improvement in motor function, but at the expense of unique complications. Newer approaches, such as gene therapy, present exciting new potential treatments. It is important to realize that early participants in surgical programs are younger, more motivated, and healthier than the PD population at large. We must begin to subject surgical studies to the same kind of rigor (including the use of comparison groups) to which we subject medical therapies. Only time will determine the ultimate role of surgical treatments of PD.

The clinician should not neglect patients' feelings of anger and loss that accompany a diagnosis of PD, particularly in those who have always 'followed the rules' and taken care of their health. Support groups, lay advocacy organizations, and other social support systems play an important role in the management of the disease. Patients and family members can access the Internet to extend their reach to support networks across the world. As physicians, listening to support and advocacy groups, as well as to our patients, will help us to continue to improve the lives of people affected by PD.

Index

NOTES